Institutionalizing Illness Narratives

Mathew George

Institutionalizing Illness Narratives

Discourses on Fever and Care from Southern India

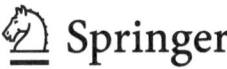 Springer

Mathew George
School of Health Systems Studies, Centre
   for Public Health
Tata Institute of Social Sciences
Mumbai, Maharashtra
India

ISBN 978-981-10-1904-3   ISBN 978-981-10-1905-0   (eBook)
DOI 10.1007/978-981-10-1905-0

Library of Congress Control Number: 2016944412

Printed on acid-free paper

This Springer imprint is published by Springer Nature
The registered company is Springer Science+Business Media Singapore Pte Ltd.

We are at grave risk of what I call "Type II Medical Malpractice"—doctors doing the unnecessary, albeit very well (as opposed to Type I Medical Malpractice, which is doctors doing the necessary unacceptably poorly). Until the public at large comes to recognize the dangers of medicalization and Type II Medical Malpractice and decries both, there will be no pressure to reform an egregiously self-serving national medical enterprise. We will continue to condemn its costliness rather than its abysmal lack of cost-effectiveness.

—Nortin M. Hadler, *Worried Sick, A Prescription for Health in an Overtreated America,* 2008, University of North Carolina Press, Chapel Hill

To Alpana

Preface

Fever as an illness or distress has occupied a prominent position in both historical and contemporary realms of medicine and society. This could be due to the fact that fevers loom large as a symptom for a range of diseases as well as in the diverse understandings prevalent about the illness. The way in which fever is perceived and understood by different societies and different groups has never been the same. Further, it is widely accepted that what one sees depends, in part, on the intellectual framework through which it is looked upon. It is this characteristic that makes fever among the more complex illnesses, where clinical identification is considered a difficult task. This is because diseases change their meaning over time as well as among societies, leading to an inability to achieve a unified understanding of fevers. The present book is about fevers, a category that has a varied understanding among different groups in Kerala society, and examines how fever care is rendered in allopathic hospitals, the dominant and extensively utilized system of medicine in the state. The book unravel the complexities involved in the understanding of fevers during the post-monsoon period in the state of Kerala where deaths due to fever are reported every year. Moreover, focussing on the role of health institutions in creating and propagating notions about illness calls for an analysis on how medical care is rendered to fever patients. This close examination of fever care helps to unravel various characteristics of medicine, as it is said that the history of fevers is also the history of medicine. This close association between fevers and medicine in historic times is also relevant in the contemporary period. Medical care in general has two different dimensions. First is the way in which a nation organizes care to its people wherein the role of public- and private-sector health care providers and the policy towards provisioning become cardinal. Second and usually less explored is the culture of medical care that examines the acts of medical practice and the production of medical knowledge, which engages with the inherent logic of reductionism as in the case of biomedicine and its confrontation with uncertainty. What the book tries to highlight more is the latter, thereby demonstrating that it becomes inevitable to examine the latter to make better sense of the former. The study uses a critical medical anthropology approach and will be a contribution to the social study of medicine, also called as medicine studies, through an inquiry into a common illness, namely fever.

Scenario of Epidemics

Epidemics during post-monsoon periods have become a normal phenomenon in India. Outbreaks of dengue, cholera, malaria, leptospirosis and chikungunya are reported from different parts of the country almost every year. Public health emergencies like epidemic outbreaks reveal the response of the state in the maintenance of public order in modern societies. Epidemics of Japanese encephalitis from Uttar Pradesh and dengue in Delhi have been reported during post-monsoon periods. In Kerala, during the post-monsoon period, fevers as a broad category, which include viral fevers, rat fever (leptospirosis), and dengue fever, together take their toll in epidemic proportions every year. In the state of Kerala, until the mid-1980s, fevers as a broad category included viral fevers, the common cold, runny nose, and other similar infections. During the late-1990s, due to increased reporting of the number of cases of rat fever, dengue fever, and viral fever in the state, a perceived threat of fevers was generated, and the distinction between the types of fever became difficult. This inability to distinguish between fevers occurred despite the fact that the state has better access to health services (both public and private) and that they are utilised extensively. The focus of the media was more on rat fever and dengue fever and the deaths due to these diseases. This was because these diseases were perceived as a new threat and because the emergence of new diseases was the talk of the day. Once the newness of the diseases subsided, the media started concentrating on deaths due to a range of fevers, resulting in the production of a new category of deaths—panimaranangal (fever deaths). It is at this juncture that the health minister of Kerala in May 2004 declared the establishment of fever clinics in all district and taluk (block) hospitals and major community health centres in the state. Fever clinics became a separate wing of the previous outpatient departments, where only fever patients were then rendered care. It is possible that the meaning attached to fever could be different for different people. For instance, fevers could be a symptom in the eyes of doctors and a state of ill health for the public, whereas for public health experts, the same could be considered an epidemic. It is in this context that the book explores the establishment of fever clinics in the state.

Context of Fever Talk

Fever talk implies the varied understandings about the illness, fever. This is based on the premise that the understanding and perception about fevers is determined by the discourses about disease, illness, and medicine, by the provisioning of health services, and the practice of medicine. Here, two aspects become important: first, the way illness/disease is seen by different groups, such as those affected, doctors or physicians, and health experts. It is obvious that for each, the purpose is different while dealing with the illness, as their understanding about the illness and their response is varied. According to Yardley, "the meaning of a word cannot therefore be adequately continued in a restrictive dictionary-style definition; meaning is not fixed but ambiguous, and so is created by the word's context and usage, including the intentions and understanding of the speaker-writer and the listener-reader" (1997: 14). Secondly, it is important to consider that individuals' lives are delimited by a combination of physical and social constraints and potentialities that can result in diverse perceptions of reality. This is because social structures such as working and housing conditions and practices such as dietary habits and health customs have as real and inevitable impacts on the health of many working-class people as do physical entities such as viruses, genes, or environmental pollutants.

Dual Dimensions of Fever Care

In order to understand fever care, the discourses on illness and disease as prevalent in the discipline of sociology of health and illness as well as in the sociology of medicine become important. It has to be noted that any attempt to understand disease/illness dichotomy has to address the question of diagnosis, which in turn, determines prognosis and treatment, which ultimately becomes the basis of medical care. Medical care is a very broad concept that encompasses a range of activities carried out by a health facility for the well-being of the people. Two aspects of medical care will be the focus of this volume. First, the text examines medical care in terms of the provisioning of treatment, which is based on the organisation of medical care, as influenced by the role of the public and private sector in a society that is either market-driven or that has a state responsibility to organise medical care for a nation. Further, the ways in which primary, secondary, and tertiary care are provided by the above sectors will also be addressed from a policy perspective. Any study on the provisioning of health services calls for a beneficiary perspective for a complete understanding. The utilisation of health services from a patient perspective becomes inevitable and is based on the concept of health-seeking behaviour where the socioeconomic and cultural milieu of the beneficiary is given due consideration. The cultural context of the society, namely the risk discourse of an epidemic and the prevalence of medicalisation becomes a precondition for understanding people's behaviour.

Secondly, the practice of medicine (culture of medical practice) within the microcosm of a clinic will be examined, as there are several micro factors that determine the behaviour of the doctor and the patient that ultimately affect the outcome of medical care. In other words, the role of medicine in society is understood through an inquiry into its practice within the context of what medicine is. This leads to the argument on the disciplinary status of medicine—whether it is an art or science or both. Going further, there are arguments that medicine is neither an art nor a science, but *tekne iatrique*, a technique of healing that is culturally shaped and thus endorses the argument that medicine is culture. Moreover, analyses from the perspective of the sociology of medical knowledge focus on the production of medical categories and how doctors and patients mediate these processes.

Here, it is well understood that doctors and patients are the major actors, especially in an acute illness like fever where doctor–patient interaction becomes cardinal, as it is through this engagement that medical work gets accomplished. Doctor–patient interaction has been an area of focus for a range of scholars who studied the sociology of profession. This book examines doctor–patient interaction as a narrative using the concept of voice.

Chapterisation

Chapter 1 traces several theoretical approaches in the field of sociology that provide appropriate frameworks for the analysis of an epidemic and how medicine interacts with society through the process of medical care. The chapter examines the changing relationship of disease and illness, the varied approaches prevalent in the relationship between medicine and society, as well as the approaches to understanding the social production of medical knowledge. A brief description of the social characteristics of Kerala society in general, and health characteristics in particular, will be carried out that will set the context for the study. Chapter 2 is about the historical discourse on fevers in the west during the eighteenth, nineteenth, and the twentieth centuries, within which the discourses in the Indian subcontinent during the nineteenth and the twentieth century are explored.

Chapter 3 contextualizes the contemporary scenario of fevers in Kerala state, especially for the post-1990s epidemic during which fever clinics were established. This will be based on examining various events that happened in the society using multi-site ethnography. The chapter demonstrates how the institutionalization of epidemics and clinics takes place in the context of a societal threat of an epidemic.

Chapter 4 examines the diverse interpretations of fever prevalent in the society among the people and the biomedical fraternity. Further, the risk discourse in public health is engaged with in the context of a fear of fevers that operates in the society. This risk discourse acquires newer meanings in the context of a medicalised society and commodification that exist as an outcome of the way medical care is organised. This is based on the analysis of the differences in nature and characteristics of care rendered by public and private hospitals and the treatment-seeking behaviour of those affected. The patient characteristics not only demonstrate diverse understandings of fevers across various groups but also their varied responses to fevers during different stages of the illness.

Chapter 5 examines fever care with a focus on its cultural dimension. This is based on the ethnography of a clinic that examines the procedures, administrative and medical, involved in fever care. In other words, this chapter deals with the processes of diagnosis, prognosis, and therapeutics involved in fever care that reveal various factors influencing the above processes and therefore the medical outcome. Through the lens of fever care, the chapter raises questions pertaining to the practice of biomedicine in the current context where medical uncertainty and the social influences of medical practice are demonstrated.

Doctor–patient interaction that is cardinal in the process of medical care is the central theme of the sixth chapter. In this chapter, doctor–patient interaction is seen as a text where two actors interact during their everyday activity in the context of the same event, illness, whose understanding could be diverse. This interaction is analysed using narrative analysis where the above context becomes cardinal.

Finally, the last chapter draws on the linkages between provisioning and medicalisation in the context of fear of fevers and demonstrates how the response to an epidemic reveals the capacity of the state in rendering medical care. It also focuses on the role of risk discourse in the context of public health practice, wherein multiple dimensions of risk are unravelled. It is in this context that medicalisation and commercialization, two important aspects of contemporary medical care, are examined and their mutual linkage is articulated. This raises some pertinent questions on what ought to be the nature of biomedical practice and its implications on people's access to medical care.

Mumbai, India   Mathew George

Reference

Yardley, L. (ed.). (1997) *Material discourses of health and illness*. London: Routledge.

Acknowledgments

Working on a book that lies in the interface of public health and medical anthropology has been a unique experience, as the very field of public health is at the crossroads where biomedical and social epidemiological approaches negotiate their pathways while responding to a public health crisis. This book is an offshoot from my doctoral thesis that interprets fever talk and fever care in the southern Indian state of Kerala, which was an outcome of an attempt to understand 'epidemic fevers' from a public health perspective. The inquiry has taken several turns and largely diverges from the field of public health in its attempt to understand and interpret the actual meaning of events as understood and experienced by the actors involved. This 'meaning-seeking' exercise has resulted in my entering the field of medical anthropology and further, the sociology of medicine, also known as medicine studies.

In the writing of this book, I owe my heartfelt gratitude to my brilliant supervisors, Dr. Alpana D. Sagar and Dr. Harish Naraindas, for their invaluable comments and contributions that not only enriched my thesis, but that also helped me understand the very art of doing research.

Dr. Alpana Sagar was a constant inspiration to me throughout my work. Her training in medicine and public health, along with her conscious efforts to situate medicine within the complexities of society, helped me to adopt a more critical approach. I am also thankful for her guidance and her sincere effort towards the development of this manuscript during her difficult times. I wish she were here to see this work finally coming to fruition.

Dr. Harish Naraindas must also be credited for his contributions, which helped shape my perspective in addressing the many facets of biomedical practice. His courses on the sociology of medicine and narrative analysis in the social sciences gave me confidence to carry out an in-depth examination of the doctor–patient interaction and the social context of medical practice, which in turn helped me tremendously in writing the last two chapters of this book. His constant encouragement was a motivation for me during the various phases of this work.

I also acknowledge the contribution of the faculty members of the Centre of Social Medicine and Community Health, School of Social Sciences, Jawaharlal Nehru University, in their diverse capacities that helped me inculcate a 'social science perspective' to public health issues, which I hope is well reflected in the book: Prof. Imrana Qadeer, for orienting me to the evolution of Indian health services that has engendered my conviction for the need for a public sector-dominated health care delivery system; Prof. K.R. Nayar, for taking us through the methodological challenges in the social sciences and their linkages to the field of public health. Prof. Rao for cautioning about the international influences in Indian Public health; Prof. Ritu Priya, for constantly reminding me of the need for a public health perspective in approaching any health problem; Prof. Rama Baru, for orienting me to the fields of medical sociology and public health, and sowing the seeds of a possible theory of illness from a social science perspective; and finally, Prof. Sangamitra Acharya, for orienting me to quantitative techniques.

The engagement with Prof. Dhruv Raina through his course on the social theory of science helped me to become familiar with approaches within the stream of social studies of science that I used in the fifth chapter. Professor Neeladri Bhattacharyya's course on historical methods contributed to my understanding of the history of Western medicine in general and fevers in particular, which was useful in developing the second chapter of this book.

For my fieldwork, I thank the government hospital authorities as well as the private institutions and the staff of these institutes for extending their support and cooperation for this study. Special mention should be made of the Directorate of Health Services (DHS), Thiruvananthapuram, and the authorities of the four health facilities selected for the study. In addition, the doctors, paramedical staff, and other staff of various health facilities require special mention, as they were highly cooperative during the data collection period despite their busy schedules.

Above all, I extend my heartfelt thanks and concern to the patients and their families who agreed to be part of the study, realizing that they themselves would not benefit directly from this study, but stood by my side for the sake of a larger cause. Words are insufficient to express my thanks, as it was during their worst times of illness that they agreed to be part of the research, and without them the study would have never been possible.

I also wish to thank various libraries in Kerala, the National Medical Library, New Delhi, and the Indian Institute of Health Management Research (IIHMR), Jaipur, for their cooperation. The main library at Jawaharlal Nehru University deserves special mention. I acknowledge the documentation unit at the Centre of Social Medicine and Community Health for the warmth of the staff members, Mrs. Rastogi, Mr. Dinesh, and Mr. Duraipandi, in providing a homely environment for my research.

I extend my sincere thanks to the Indian Council of Social Science Research (ICSSR) for the financial assistance provided for the completion of the study.

Above all, there is the kind of JNU life that made this study happen in the present form. I want to mention the tea sessions and subsequent discussions of everything on earth that have been a feature of hostel life, which I am sure has contributed not only to the making of the book but to my own self as well.

Special thanks go to my friends at JNU, both the old and new generation, for their support in various capacities. Bandar, a left collective for Kerala studies formed during my last years at JNU, was not only an emotional inspiration but also reasserted the urgent need to approach the problems of Kerala society from a different perspective.

At the Tata Institute of Social Sciences, Mumbai, where I have been working as faculty of the School of Health Systems Studies, I would like to thank my students who have questioned me and helped me to sharpen my arguments. Special thanks go to my faculty colleagues for creating an environment in which to discuss the varied meanings of medical care and public health.

Special mention must be made of the opportunity to develop a course on medical anthropology and public health as part of my pre-doctoral teaching, in which there was close engagement with the risk discourse in public health and medical practice, which helped in developing the fourth chapter in its current form

I would like to extend my wholehearted thanks to my parents and siblings for their unfailing support and critical engagement in whatever I do in my life. Last but not the least, I owe so much to my wife, Ailoo, and my children, Naveen and Nanditha, for supporting me every day, even when I fail to give adequate time both as a husband and a father.

A book is always the result of the contributions of several people in various capacities, both intellectual and otherwise. I thank the Springer publishing team, especially the editorial team, Ms. Shinjini Chatterjee and Ms. Shruti Raj, for their sincere and meticulous efforts throughout the publishing process. At this juncture I acknowledge all those contributions that made this work possible, though some of these contributions I may not even realize. I alone am responsible for any shortcomings in this work.

Mathew George

Contents

1 **Interpreting Illness, Disease, Medicine, and Medical Care** 1
  1.1   Introduction 1
  1.2   The Concept of Disease: The Philosophical Debate 2
  1.3   Sociologists' Approach to Illness and Disease 4
      1.3.1   Sick Role 5
      1.3.2   Illness Behaviour to Illness 5
      1.3.3   Disease as Culturally Defined 6
  1.4   Medicine and Society 8
  1.5   Interpreting Medicine 11
  1.6   Medical Care as Provisioning and Culture 12
  1.7   The Sociology of Medical Knowledge 13
  1.8   The Study 16
  1.9   The Setting 17
      1.9.1   Social Development in Kerala 17
      1.9.2   Kerala's Morbidity and Health Care Scenario 18
      1.9.3   The Hospital Setting 19
  1.10   Theoretical Framework 20
  1.11   Secondary-Level Hospitals: The District Hospital
       and the Immanuel Hospital 22
  1.12   Public Hospital at the Primary Level: Community
       Health Centre 22
  1.13   Sivani Hospital 23
  1.14   Commonalties and Differences in Hospital Procedures 23
  1.15   'Being a Participant Observer' 24
  References 25

2 **Historical Discourses on Fevers** 29
  2.1   Introduction 29
  2.2   Early History of Fevers in the West 30
  2.3   Classification of Fevers 31

2.4   Fevers During the Sixteenth and Seventeenth Centuries:
      Descriptive to Problematic 32
2.5   Practising Physicians' Knowledge of Fevers:
      An Eighteenth-Century Characteristic.................... 33
2.6   Classification of Fevers: The Primary Task During the
      Early Nineteenth Century 34
2.7   Morgagni and 'Pathological Anatomy' 36
2.8   Late Nineteenth- and Early Twentieth-Century
      Pathologisation on Fever. 38
2.9   History of Fevers in the Indian Subcontinent. 39
2.10 History of Public Health in Travancore. 42
      2.10.1 International Interventions in Public Health.......... 43
2.11 Medical Care in Travancore 43
      2.11.1 Fevers in Travancore 44
      2.11.2 Fever Care in Twentieth-Century Kerala. 45
2.12 History of Fevers and Public Health. 46
References 47

3 **Institutionalising Fever Epidemics and Fever Care
   in Contemporary Kerala** 49
   3.1   Fevers as Discourse 49
   3.2   Discourse Analysis as Theory and Method 50
   3.3   Disease Profile of Contemporary Kerala 52
         3.3.1 Epidemic Fevers 52
         3.3.2 Reporting Fevers 55
   3.4   Fever Talk: The Discursive Production of a Disease. 56
         3.4.1 Response from the Media and the Public 57
         3.4.2 Fever Talk in Plural Systems of Medicine. 59
         3.4.3 Establishment of Fever Clinics 60
   3.5   Fever Clinics at Work 62
         3.5.1 Biomedical Practice 63
         3.5.2 Transactions in a Fever Clinic 63
         3.5.3 The Process of Diagnosis 64
   3.6   Discourses on Institutionalising an Epidemic. 66
   References 67

4 **Fear of Fevers: Risk, Medicalisation, and Provisioning** 69
   4.1   Introduction 69
   4.2   Selection of Patients. 71
   4.3   Health-Seeking Behaviour. 71
   4.4   Interpreting Fevers in Kerala. 73
         4.4.1 Fever as that Which Interrupts Day-to-Day Life. 73
         4.4.2 Tracing the Causes. 74
         4.4.3 Fever: During and After Suffering 75

4.5   Biomedical Interpretation of *Fevers*   76
4.6   Lay Versus Medical Categorisation   78
        4.6.1   Perceiving Fevers.   79
        4.6.2   Response to Fevers   81
        4.6.3   Time of Seeking Treatment.   83
        4.6.4   Number of Hospitals Visited Per Episode   84
        4.6.5   Interpreting Illness Behaviour   84
4.7   Provisioning of Medical Care   85
4.8   Fever Care as Provisioning.   87
        4.8.1   Nature of Provisioning of Fever Care: A Population
                  Perspective   88
        4.8.2   Fever Care in Hospitals   89
        4.8.3   Extent of Laboratory Tests   90
        4.8.4   Total Medical Expenditure for One
                  Episode of Fever   91
4.9   Heterogeneity in Private-Sector Health Care   93
4.10   Commercialisation of Fever Care.   94
4.11   Risk, Medicalisation, and Provisioning.   94
References   96

5   **Biomedicine Examined: Interpreting the Culture of Fever Care**. ...   99
5.1   Introduction   99
5.2   Early History of Biomedicine   100
5.3   Lineage of Contemporary Biomedicine.   102
        5.3.1   Contemporary Biomedical Practice.   106
5.4   Culture of Medical Practice.   107
        5.4.1   Culture of Fever Care.   108
5.5   Medical Record: A Vehicle for Accomplishing
        Medical Work.   109
5.6   Diagnosis in Biomedicine.   111
        5.6.1   Ethnography of Diagnosis.   113
        5.6.2   Medical Uncertainty Despite Laboratory
                  Investigations   115
        5.6.3   Vanishing Thermometers in Fever Clinics.   116
        5.6.4   Body Temperature Versus Erythrocyte
                  Sedimentation Rate (ESR).   118
5.7   Treatment Modalities   120
        5.7.1   Symptomatic Treatment   121
        5.7.2   Demonstrating Macro Influences Within the
                  Microcosm of Medical Work.   123
5.8   Societal Discourse of an Epidemic Interferes
        with Fever Care.   124
        5.8.1   Preventive Diagnostics for Surveillance:
                  Expanding Functions of Hospitals   125

          5.8.2   Moral Hazard: Insurance Coverage as a Driver
                  of Hospital Admission   127
     5.9   Fever Care as Sub-culture of Biomedicine   127
     References   129

6   **Voice of Illness and Voice of Medicine in
     Doctor–Patient Interaction**   131
     6.1   Introduction   132
     6.2   Understanding the Doctor–Patient Interaction   132
     6.3   Narratives and the Social World   134
     6.4   Narrative Analysis of the Doctor–Patient Interaction.   135
     6.5   Situating Institutions in Illness Narratives   135
     6.6   Narrative as a Mode of Communication:
            Voices of Interaction   136
     6.7   Voice(s) of Medicine   137
     6.8   The Context   138
     6.9   Voice of Illness   139
     6.10   Medicalised Voice and Voice(s) of Medicine   142
     6.11   Therapeutic Interaction: A Site of Knowledge Production   144
     6.12   Interaction of *Thought Styles*   145
     References   147

7   **Fever Talk as a Sub-culture of Fever Care**   149
     7.1   Medical Care and Medical Practice   155
     7.2   The Way Forward   156

Glossary   159

Bibliography   161

About the Author

Mathew George, MPH, Ph.D. is Assistant Professor and Chairperson of the Centre for Public Health, School of Health Systems Studies, Tata Institute of Social Sciences, Mumbai. His training is in public health, with a doctorate in social medicine and community health from Jawaharlal Nehru University (JNU), New Delhi. His research interest is in the field of sociology of health and illness, with special emphasis on the sociology of medical practice and medical knowledge in biomedicine, and on the interaction between multiple systems of medicine. He is currently working on the scope of introducing a public health cadre into the Indian health services system from a social epidemiological perspective.

Abbreviations

AIDS	Acquired immune deficiency syndrome
ARI	Acute respiratory infection
BPL	Below poverty line
CHC	Community health centre
COPD	Chronic obstructive pulmonary disorder
DHS	Directorate of Health Services
DLHS	District-level household survey
DMO	District medical officer
ECG	Electrocardiography
ELISA	Enzyme-linked immunosorbent assay
ENT	Ear, nose, throat
ESR	Erythrocyte sedimentation rate
GP	General practitioner
HMO	Health maintenance organisation
ICU	Intensive care unit
IEC	Information, education, and communication
IgG	Immunoglobulin G
IgM	Immunoglobulin M
IIPS	International Institute for Population Sciences
IMA	Indian Medical Association
IP	Inpatient
IV fluid	Intravenous fluid
JE	Japanese encephalitis
KKK	Kai kal kodachal
KSSP	Kerala Sastra Sahitya Parishad
LMS	London Mission Society
LRTI	Lower respiratory tract infection
MAT	Microscopic agglutination test
MCH	Medical college hospital
ME	Migrant employee

MICU	Medical intensive care unit
NSSO	National Sample Survey Organisation
OBC	Other backward caste
OEC	Other eligible caste
OGHMOK	Organisation of Government Homoeo Medical Officers Kerala
OP	Outpatient
PHC	Primary health centre
PUO	Pyrexia of unknown origin
RCH	Reproductive and child health
SAT	Sri Avittom Thirunal
SC	Scheduled caste
SES	Socio-economic status
SLI	Standard of life index
ST	Scheduled tribe
TAB	Typhoid vaccine A and B
TB	Tuberculosis
TSB	Treatment-seeking behaviour
URTI	Upper respiratory tract infection
UTI	Urinary tract infection
VD	Venereal disease
WBC	White blood cells
WHO	World Health Organisation

Chapter 1
Interpreting Illness, Disease, Medicine, and Medical Care

Abstract The concept of disease is understood differently by philosophers, sociologists, and biomedical professionals, a reality that becomes obvious when one examines the concept across disciplines. A close examination of its linkage with medicine reveals the reciprocal relationship of medicine and society, and thereby highlights the power of medicine to control society through its categories, namely disease. The present chapter explores the diverse nature of our understanding of disease across disciplines, in order to interpret the role of medicine in society. It also examines how medical care is organised, particularly in terms of its provisioning, as an outcome of governmental policies with respect to health care and its culture of medical practice, wherein the doctor–patient interaction becomes pivotal, as it is through this interaction that an inquiry into the sociology of medical knowledge becomes possible. This interaction and linkage is conceptualised within the local context of Kerala society, with its unique characteristics that make the relationship more dynamic and, at times, critical. Thus, from a critical medical anthropology perspective, it becomes the task of the sociologist and anthropologist to recognise *all* knowledge—scientific, medical, and cultural—that is socially produced within a given setting. This task is amplified upon close examination of the major actors in the practice of medical care that takes place within the networks of the clinic.

Keywords Illness · Disease · Culture of medical practice · Medical knowledge · Medicalisation · Medicine studies

1.1 Introduction

The concepts of illness and disease become cardinal in any attempt to understand disease and epidemics in society. This is because disease itself is understood differently by philosophers, sociologists, and biomedical professionals, which becomes obvious when one examines the concept across disciplines. Furthermore, the close examination of its linkage with medicine not only reveals the reciprocal relationship between medicine and society but also highlights the power of medicine to control society through its categories, such as disease. The present chapter explores these diverse facets of understanding diseases across disciplines in order to interpret medicine's role in society. Additionally, how medical care is organised within a society will be focussed on in terms of its provisioning, and the way that medicine is practised in a given setting will be explored through the culture of medical practice. In this discussion, the former is revealed as mostly an outcome of government policies with respect to health care while the latter must be situated within the larger context of societal engagement with medicine and therefore medical culture. Moreover, within the culture of medical practice it is the doctor–patient interaction that becomes pivotal, not only because it can authenticate notions of disease and illness as interpreted by medicine but also due to the fact that it is through this interaction that many of the lay categories of illness get transformed to that of medicine, thereby opening a channel for inquiry into the sociology of medical knowledge.

1.2   The Concept of Disease: The Philosophical Debate

The concept of disease is a complex area that has been dealt with by several scholars in the fields of medicine and humanities, both of which fail to offer an adequate explanation. Due to the diverse nature of disease, it is very difficult to create a uniform set of criteria defining the concept that can be made applicable to all known prevalent diseases. Historically, the concept of disease was never static and universal, as reflected in the seventeenth-century categorisation by Thomas Sydenham that attributed the notion of *being* to disease, based on class and species. Later, the opening up of corpses resulted in the prominence of *site* in disease definition and subsequent shifts to include the distortion of *function* of human organs (Cartwright 1977; Reiser 1978; Foucault 1975). Furthermore, by the mid-nineteenth century, Claude Bernard treated disease (as a pathological state) as the exaggeration, disproportion, or discordance of the normal phenomena. Finally, the contribution of Virchow's cell theory and Koch's germ theory emphasised the importance of an aetiological agent in disease explanation. Thus, the evolution of disease categorisation can be seen as based initially on anatomical lesions, then on functional disturbances, and finally, on the presence of micro-organisms. Therefore, the current context of disease classification follows a mixture of these varied approaches depending on the type of disease (Wulff 1990).

In addition to the above, debates over disease definition involved whether one should define it based on bodily distress (somatic) alone or that of a combination of mental distress (psycho) together with the role of environment, both physical and social. This latter aspect offers normative explanations, which argue that disease has to be defined contextually according to a society's norms (Brown 1985). The issue of whether disease is a matter of somatic or mental distress or both is only an extension of the mind–body problem in philosophy, which was later resolved by offering a solution that considers disease as psychosomatic. However, the biomedical model further reduces its mechanistic model of disease definition as that which deviates from the norm of measurable biological (somatic) variables where the reasons for behavioural aberrations are also searched on the basis of disordered somatic processes (Engel 1977). Another problem that was mentioned earlier is that of statistical normality, which again is perceived as a value-neutral and therefore *scientific* concept. In actual situations, normality is largely based on a society's existing norm, and thus may shift with the changing nature of society and medicine (Brown 1985). This contextual aspect embedded in the definition of disease is acknowledged by Engel (1977: 132), who thereby proposes a *biopsychosocial* model of disease that envisages the need to address the social, psychological, and biological aspects that take into account (1) the patient, (2) the social context in which one lives, and (3) the contemporary systems devised by a society to deal with the disruptive effects of illness. It is this contextual nature of diseases that Rosenberg (1989) highlights when he says that the framing of disease or its defi- nition during the past as well as in the contemporary period is a complex activity, both influenced by culture and vice versa. He further argues that there is a need to examine the role of the state in defining and responding to disease and more importantly to the organisation of the medical profession and institutional medical care, specifically as a response to particular patterns of disease incidence.

Ananth (2008) in his recent book examined Boorse's (1976) concept of disease,[1] which is rooted in statistical abnormality and pathological conditions and is based on 'part function'. Here, it is important to note that pathology itself is based on statistical abnormality and pathological condition of a part or parts of the body that may or may not disrupt the overall functioning of the body. There could also be situations where statistical normality does not lead to functional normality, in which the role of context becomes cardinal. This contradiction becomes severe when one examines the difference that exists between the pathologist's view of disease and the physician's view. In other words, who should have the authority to define disease: a physician, a philosopher, or a pathologist? This led to the analysis of the field of pathology and their contributions to disease definitions for which there is no consensus. This is because pathologists do not consistently agree on the functional attributes of various parts of organisms, and thus making a judgement about the right function is difficult to say the least. The critique by Canguilhem (1991) of the

---

[1]Christopher Boorse is a strong proponent of the naturalist strand of thought, which is still the dominant paradigm in the field despite criticisms by normativists. Boorse distinguishes value-ladenness in the concept of disease by arguing that there are two versions of disease definition, namely one that follows the theory of biology, considered to be more 'scientific' and free from any values and the latter following the theory of clinicians, based on the value of clinicians and the patient's context. This raises the question of who is the right person to categorise a person's disease. Per Boorse, it should be the biologist, which in the current context should be the laboratory investigators, and the physiologists who should be defining disease theoretically, while the doctors' role is secondary and value-based. H. Tristam Engelhardt, Jr., one of the strong proponents in the normativist camp on the concept of health, strongly counters Boorse's position by arguing that the value-ladenness and contextual nature of disease definition is inevitable; for more details, see Ananth (2008).

discipline of pathology with regard to normality is a point that informs this debate. This is especially significant in the current context of laboratory medicine, where within a culture of technology-induced medicalisation, a greater tendency to define disease in the pathologists' way is implicit in the dominant discourse.

Further, the way in which Boorse has understood biology as a discipline is questioned on two accounts. First, based on evolutionary perspective in biology all species are evolving and as such, so are their functions. Boorse counters this by arguing that his standard of function refers to a specific spatiotemporal context, thereby justifying the fact that disease categories and definitions can change over time and thus must be analysed within their relevant contexts (Ananth 2008). Another criticism of the nature of biology is its failure to acknowledge the environment, which strongly influences the notion of abnormality in disease definitions. In general, statistical abstractions that define normality fail to take into account the context of environment that essentially determines whether something is normal or abnormal. A departure from the above two criticisms is that the concept of disease is more theoretical and value-free, and hence has little to do with medical practice. Rather, medicine treats the concept of disease within a given context in order to make decisions, in which case it is the context that matters—for example, the type of work, the age of the patient, and the family characteristics. One can argue that medicine is practised not necessarily like a scientific activity similar to that of a laboratory but is instead guided by existing scientific categories such as disease, which are in turn a product of medical practice. This adherence to scientific categories while practicing medicine may reduce uncertainties and abuse of the technical aspects within medicine. Still, it must be noted that the concept of disease as it is used in the current context, dominant at least in the field of biomedical practice, hovers around its *scientificity* and value neutrality, which constitutes a serious debate in the field of sociology of health and illness (George 2014a).

1.3   Sociologists' Approach to Illness and Disease

Given the complexities prevalent in the definition of disease within philosophy, it is astonishing that no serious attempt was made to examine the concept of disease per se in the field of sociology during early times. Disease was historically taken for granted as existing within the terrain of the natural sciences, thereby introducing illness as *disease plus meaning*, using Atkinson's (1995: 24) terminology where illness became part of meaning, province, and understanding that were the terrain of sociologists. Thus, sociologists largely confined themselves to the analysis of illness behaviour and the *sick role*, until more recently, when the constructivists started questioning the core categories of medicine (Sujatha 2014). A brief overview on the above concepts are dealt with below, giving due consideration to the ways in which the concepts of disease and illness have been approached from different perspectives.

1.3.1 Sick Role

It was Parsons' *sick role* that became a persuasive perspective for sociologists to use in examining patient behaviour during distress. The *sick role* is conceptualised as a counterpart to the practitioner's role, where both are part of the social system of medical practice (Parsons 1951). He further elaborates the *sick role* as characterised by two rights and two obligations. The former includes the right to receive, at least to a certain degree and for a certain time, a regular income and regular support without earning or deserving them. Second, the sick will plead for their present state, as they are considered unfit to take responsibility for their own actions. These rights lead to two obligations. The first is to recover quickly, not at their own capacity but with the non-sick environment. The second is to seek treatment and participate to the best of their ability in the treatment process until they are freed from sickness and therefore from the sick role (Parsons 1951: 436–437; Gerhardt 1987). The sick role concept has to be appreciated for its initial attempt to understand patient behaviour, attitude, and belief at the time of distress. On the other hand, it has been widely criticised for its failure to explain diversities among patients with mental and chronic illnesses, as many of these conditions do not necessarily have a cure for the associated distress that they cause, along with the fact that there exist considerable differences in cultural notions of diseases, care, and cure (Mechanic 1969; Kleinman et al. 1978; Gerhardt 1987). Another criticism has been that it is premised on a medico-centric perspective that overestimates the therapeutic impact of the physician and medical institutions (Sujatha 2014). This critique is derived from the Parsonian view of illness as deviance and health as a process of adaptation implicit in its conception, as it may ignore (though it does not deny) the capacity of humans within the physical and sociocultural environment (Gallagher 1976). Despite all of the above, Parsons' contribution remained the basis for a range of scholars in their initial understanding of health behaviour and later health-seeking behaviour, and therefore traces of their understanding of the concepts of illness and disease can be seen even now.

1.3.2 Illness Behaviour to Illness

Owing to the introduction of the *sick role,* a host of scholars have studied illness behaviour and health-seeking behaviour, of whom Mechanic (1969), Suchman (1963), and Kasl and Cobb (1966) are a few. It was through the definition of illness behaviour and an understanding of its nature that the concept of illness subsequently was established. Thus, illness was broadly defined as any response in terms of a personal, interpersonal, or cultural reaction to disease or discomfort by an individual. Disease was defined as a malfunctioning or maladaptation of biologic and psycho-physiologic processes in an individual (Mechanic 1969; Kasl and Cobb 1966). Many scholars retained a similar kind of distinction between illness and disease in which disease was given a physiological, universal, taken-for-granted status whereas illness was the accepted domain of analysis for sociologists. Though a sociological concept, illness was seen by some scholars as having an individualistic connotation, as it is substituted by 'sickness' since the latter addresses the social context more pronouncedly (Young 1982). A different take on the path to conceptualising illness and disease occurred when Kleinman et al. (1978) began to approach medical systems as cultural systems where illness was considered as important and necessary to understanding disease in its totality. This in a way critiqued the notion of disease as a natural *entity*. Instead, disease was seen as belonging to culture, that being the specialised culture of medicine. In this view, culture is not only a means of representing disease, but is essential to its very constitution as a human reality (Kleinman 1980).

1.3.3 Disease as Culturally Defined

This understanding was carried forward by scholars who viewed the medical understanding of diseases as

> … the doctors' subjective, culturally-bound assessment of the reality of their patients' illness, based on a mixture of empirical observations and theoretical inter-subjective negotiated and ideological knowledge of the actors, viz. doctors and patients. It is the doctors' knowledge and interpretation of those objects and events (thought style) he comes across and the way he constitutes objects and events that he believes intelligible to other actors with whom he interacts. (Young 1981: 379–380)

Finally, the doctor produces knowledge by negotiating meaning while interacting with patients. This approach of seeing medical knowledge not as a universal, independent reality but as a participant in the construction of reality situates both illness, and more importantly, disease as concepts that are known and interpreted via social activity. This approach therefore calls for an examination of these concepts using cultural and social analysis (Sujatha 2014; Lupton 1994: 12).

One of the criticisms of sociologists to the above approach is that it is a limited view of scientific beliefs, justifying that many clinical conditions remain the same over a long period. This is to say that many of the old clinical entities can be found and felt among patients even today, though the meaning attached to them might have varied or is in a process of change. In order to make clear the above aspect,

King's (1982: 149) concept of *clinical entity*[2] and *disease entity*[3] as cited by Turner (2000) seems to be appropriate. The former is explained as a configuration or pattern that is observed by a doctor in interaction with a patient, while the latter is the knowledge about a condition that is produced by doctors' observations, statistical information, and laboratory tests. Going further, he opines that clinical entity remains relatively constant whereas disease entity is subject to change, which in turn can alter the clinical entity. This appears as an attempt to substitute the earlier position of disease entity by a new category, *clinical entity,* as if it is free of social and cultural contexts and is therefore *natural.* Turner (2000) extends his argument that a clinical reality is present and has been dealt with by physicians over centuries, which at any point of time is subject to change within the quest for new forms of knowledge. This quest in turn is influenced by general social values and changing social circumstances in which doctors are trained to recognise the signs and symptoms that announce the presence of the clinical reality. The physician's action based on his or her understanding of the clinical reality must be seen as the product of specific and local medical cultures.

Thus, it will be argued, disease or distress is a social reality that derives its meaning and relevance from a given socio-political, cultural, and historical context. These clinical and disease entities are socially produced in a given setting of medical systems whose relevance and meaning will vary for different contexts. An understanding of clinical as well as disease entities varies according to the system of medicine practised, the social groups to which the patients and the physicians belong, and more importantly, the prevalent notions about health, illness, and cure in that society (Sujatha 2014). For example, to say that *fever* is socially produced is not to say that it is a *fiction*, or that it does not exist, or that it could be treated merely as a doctor's imagination. However, the signs and symptoms of fever in a clinical setting are mediated through and by the experiences and training of physicians, and these physicians are the products of specific and local medical cultures. Above all, there is widespread agreement that conceptions of disease have

---

[2]A clinical entity is a pattern that is observed by a doctor during the bedside interaction with the patient. A disease entity is knowledge about a condition that is produced by doctors' observations, statistical information, and laboratory tests. Disease entity follows clinical entity, and thus, clinical entity is considered relatively constant. This is again an essentialist position that says there is a core that never changes and is objective. For details, *see* King (1982): 149. A similar kind of distinction is made by Boorse when he replies to moral normativists on the value–neutrality of health. He makes a distinction between theories of science of biology and practical clinical judgements made by practitioners, where the former is considered value–free and the latter value –laden. For more details, see Ananth (2008).

[3]'Disease entity' implies a combination of characteristics denoting the state of a patient, usually a product of medical diagnosis expressed as a combination of the symptoms of the patient, laboratory investigations, and psychosocial behavior valued against the social norms, which thus attain meaning and legitimacy in the social world. According to Rosenberg (2002) this transformation of disease states is a product of the changing nature of medicine thanks to the development of pathological anatomy and supportive medical technology, a feature identified since the early twentieth century. Philosophers of medicine use 'disease state' to denote this, see Engelhardt, Jr. (1976).

changed radically over a period of time (Rosenberg 1989). Not only have the conceptions changed but also the domain of analysis of disease has changed from a lay category to that of a medical category. This is to say that disease, once defined as 'dis-ease' or the expression of any distress or un-wellness of the body, was predominantly a lay category (Kraupl Taylor 1980). Later, disease became a domain of medicine where as a concept it now encompasses a range of *objective* medical categories. It is worthwhile at this juncture to examine the role of the concept of *illness*, a sociological category, in facilitating the above transformation of disease as a category to one belonging to a medical domain. Besides, taking into consideration the complexities and heterogeneity involved in disease entities (acute, chronic, mental illnesses, etc.), it would be unwise to search for a general theory of *disease* applicable to all disease entities. Instead, an approach is needed that helps us to understand *disease entity* in its totality within a specific context.

1.4 Medicine and Society

The role of medicine in society has been an object of inquiry by a range of scholars from anthropology, history, and sociology as well as from the discipline of medicine itself. This could be due to an acknowledgement of the inevitable role that medicine has in any society, as it can define and redefine our understanding of illness, disease, the body, and what constitutes normal and abnormal, both from a normative perspective as well as among the proponents of *scientific rationality*. This power of medicine to name and categorise distress, including its capacity to enter into the daily lives of human beings in order to define and redefine what ought to be the way of life, has been theorised by several scholars (Parsons 1951; Illich 1976; Foucault 1975), despite the fact that their approaches towards the nature of medicine vary considerably. The present section is an attempt to examine this nature of medicine as dealt with by various scholars while examining its impact on society.

As mentioned before, Parsons' conceptualisation of the sick role was an outcome of his attempt to understand the patient's role in contrast to the physician's role. Here, medicine is understood as comprising organised procedures premised on *scientific* and *objective* knowledge together with technical competence capable of dealing with the patient's illness/disease, through all of which the physician's attitude is seen *altruistic* (Parsons 1951: 447–454). Not only is medicine seen as capable of responding to illness, but the patient is also expected to abide by the rules of medicine set by the physician. The *altruistic* nature of the physician and the ability of medicine to cure several illnesses have been widely critiqued (Zola 1972; Illich 1976; Ehrenreich 1978). Friedson (1970), who has approached medicine from a 'profession' perspective, invokes the power of medicine through its ability to 'label' a disease, thereby exerting social control as do other institutions like the Church, rule of law, and so on. Unlike Parsons, who examines role of the patient against that of the physician, Friedson examines the physician role (*clinical mentality*) per se by situating the

physician within the sociocultural context of medical fraternity (ibid.). This professional power of medicine, he argues, is irrespective of the power of medicine to
effectively deal with the illness. Going one step further, Zola (1972) elaborates upon
the ways in which medicine as a social institution exerts control over a society. He
identifies this control in four ways: (i) the expansion of what in life is deemed relevant
to the good practice of medicine, (ii) through the retention of absolute control over
certain technical procedures, (iii) through the retention of near-absolute access to
certain 'taboo' areas (for example, pregnancy, once regarded as a normal natural
process, has later come to be seen as a 'medical problem'), and (iv) through the
expansion of what in medicine is deemed relevant to the good practice of life. This
implies medicine's power to collect minute details regarding patients' lives and to
expose patients to technical procedures as and when required, thereby restricting the
behaviour of patients in the name of good practice of life necessary for the better
practice of medicine. It is through this process that society is gradually transformed
into a medicalised society whose manifestations are a dependence on drugs and
medical care as well as increasing rates of *clinical entities* (abnormalities) in populations. The reasons for such medicalisation could be due to a combination of medicine's professional upper hand over lay interpretations of health, body, and illness,
and a basic human desire to make one feel, look, or function better (ibid.).

Ivan Illich (1976) identified medicine as a nemesis and its practice in society as
that which leads to *clinical, social* and *structural iatrogenesis*. He deals with
medicalisation slightly differently and disagrees with the ability of medicine to cure.
Instead, Illich argues that the practice of modern medicine can lead to clinical side
effects (*clinical iatrogenesis*) whose impacts may not be precipitated even in the
early stages of therapy. Second, he uses the term *social iatrogenesis* where, similar
to Zola's explanation of the *medicalisation of society,* he cautions that medical
practice will result in dependence on care and drugs, and will ultimately take away
the life of the patient. Going one step further than Zola, Illich sees the process of
medicalisation as that which is both retained by and a product of a capitalist society
(ibid. 31–66). Last, he talks about *structural iatrogenesis* where a silencing of other
systems of medicine and cultural practices occurs along with the silencing of the
body's ability to adapt to pain and ultimately to natural death (ibid. 87–120).

From a political economy perspective, it is argued that those who are ill, disabled,
aged, female, and members of other vulnerable groups suffer from poor health since
access to health care services will be restricted based on the notion that they *(the
deprived)* contribute less to the production and consumption of commodities (Navarro
1975). This can lead to institutions of medicine perpetuating social inequalities rather
than ameliorating them. The widening of medical jurisdiction over the years due to
increased medicalisation has left little scope for some patients to question its activities
or use of resources. This is considered to be due to two reasons. First, the Western
medical encounter led to the dominance of the corporate and middle class in positions
of influence in the medical system over the lower middle class and working class. The
latter comprises the bulk of patients and lesser skilled workers in the health care
system, with little control over their medical treatment or work conditions (Waitzkin
1979). Second, as part of the commodification of health care, the relationship between

doctors and patients is characterised by conflict and a clash of differing interests and priorities (Navarro 1986).

Medicine is understood as exerting power in society through the process of objectification and rationalisation (Bury 1998). This is obvious from medicine's power to categorise disease in a *scientific* way through the emergence of pathological anatomy, thereby transforming illness—a lived experience—into the domain of medicine as a disease entity. This was accomplished through the opening up of clinics where the *docile body* was subjected to the *gaze* of medicine through the powerful expertise of the profession (Foucault 1975: 107–120). It is this power of medicine that has reached a stage of surveying the population in terms of patterns of disease and abnormality, thereby subjecting society to continuous scrutiny. This rationalisation process based on statistical calculations and rigorous predictions led to what Armstrong (1995) called *surveillance medicine.* It is this process of objectification and rationalisation that has made medicine *modern* in its approach and practice. Foucault's acknowledgement of the power that medicine exerts in a society through its categories has ultimately led to a range of studies that inquire as to the possibilities of an alternative. This has brought about the critique of a range of medical categories that were historically taken for granted; thereby the biomedical category emerged as one among several frameworks through which to explain the realities located in its social and historical context (Lupton 1994; Atkinson 1995; Good 1994).

A brief discussion of the above approaches will help to identify the possibilities and pitfalls of each perspective. The process of medicalisation that generates social control is true even in the contemporary context, where dependence on drugs and care can be a feature of current biomedical practice. The political economy approach is criticised for its overemphasis on commodity nature, and thereby fails to understand the micro-social aspects of the doctor–patient relationship. Additionally, the power of medicine is seen predominantly as an outcome of professionalisation, thereby conforming to a use/abuse model[4] of medical knowledge, which in turn nullifies the alternative ways of thinking about the truth claims of biomedicine (Lupton 1994: 10). In other words, rather than identifying the problems of the biomedical model itself, the problem of medicine is seen as the way it is practised, with physicians having the upper hand and a monopoly on medical knowledge. Foucault-inspired approaches to medicine later opened up possibilities for both: issues of commodification of medicine as well as the power of medicine to *categorise,* which could catalyse the former.

---

[4]The use/abuse model is understood as such that the problems in science are due to the bad practice of it, usually attributed to the 'social' context, leaving aside the core of science, its principles, which are usually treated as 'technical'. The latter are always given a taken-for-granted status, which is rarely examined by sociologists. This model is extensively critiqued by Latour through one of his pioneering works that examined the linkages and interactions between 'social' and 'technical' in constructing a scientific fact. For more details, see Latour and Woolgar (1986).

This possibility allows the incorporation of political economy concerns, as well as the social constructionist interest in identification and labelling of disease and the meaning of illness experience (Lupton 1994: 12).

1.5   Interpreting Medicine

It is astonishing to find that while the role of biomedicine in society has been dealt with extensively by various scholars, only a few have examined the question: what *is* medicine? In other words, it becomes necessary to examine the nature and characteristics of biomedicine per se while attempting to understand its implications for society. This question was dealt with only by a few scholars, mostly philosophers, and a few others from an ethics perspective in an effort to explain what medicine *ought to be*. A brief overview of some of these reveals an attempt to grapple with the complexity of *medicine* itself. The foundational understanding of medicine then becomes critical since the notion of medicine shapes every facet of medical enterprise—the educational, the practical, the ethical, as well as the social and economic. Thus, it is possible that medicine can be approached as a discipline from an academic perspective as well as a profession (institution) based on everyday experience. From a disciplinary perspective, the question is whether medicine is a *science* or an *art*. To address this, it is important to describe what medicine is. Here, quoting Pellegrino and Thomasma (1981: 69):

Medicine is the cognitive art of applying science and persuasion through a complex human interaction in which the uniqueness of values and disease, and the kind of institution in which care is delivered, determine the nature of the judgements made"

This explanation of medicine situates clinical interaction as the core of medicine and the restoration of wellbeing as its goal. The centrality of clinical interaction allows medicine to take up several forms, as a discipline as well as a profession. Now going back to the earlier question of science and art, it is true that medicine cannot be reduced to physics, chemistry, or biology—rather, it can be derived from these sciences. While medicine does not resemble the fine arts in its products, it does share with the arts the characteristic of productive reasoning towards practical ends. This is why *medicine is treated as the most scientific of the humanities and the most humane of the sciences* (Pellegrino and Thomasma 1981: 61). Further, it is interesting to note that medicine as a solitary discipline is neither a science nor an art but owes to both. This is despite the fact that medicine and science have such a close relationship that it is necessary to investigate whether medicine has not merged with science or might not be expected to do so eventually. Munson (1981) identified certain problems in the process of medicine being identified with science. *First*, the social function of medicine to treat and prevent diseases becomes secondary to the quest for knowledge. *Second*, the practice of medicine too often under the pressure of time and immediate need tends to base decisions about intervention based on purely empirical probabilistic generalisations rather than grounded in fundamental biological processes. *Third*, physicians often consider the introduction of humanitarian ethics into medicine as something forced upon them by society or by law. Instead, the activities and aims of the discipline that are founded upon its uniqueness should generate the ethical need by itself.

Like other professions, medicine shares the dual requirements of sufficient skill and commitment to human purpose (Pellegrino and Thomasma 1981; Friedson 1970). The skill calls for a theoretical knowledge of the sciences and a creative handling of symbols such as disease and experience in applying both to the individuals. It is at this juncture that the important relationship between a physician and the patient becomes relevant. The centrality of clinical interaction reappears here as it ensures four modes of relationship: responsibility, trust, decision orientation, and aetiology, which are the elements for a successful medical event (Pellegrino and Thomasma 1981: 65–69). This is because clinical interaction involves two personal intentions that both involve a curative event—, one to seek help and the other to extend it. The above characteristics thus establish medicine as a *tekne iatrike,* a technique of healing, using Pellegrino and Thomasma's terminology. *Tekne* means knowledge of how to act according to what is the case and why it is the case (Pellegrino and Thomasma 1981). Thus, medicine is a craft that involves healing the body with the body. A simplified definition could be 'a relation of mutual consent to effect individualised well-being by working in, with and through the body' (Pellegrino and Thomasma 1981: 73). The above description of medicine seems to be an ideal case where the focus is on what *ought to be* rather than what actually *is* medicine. This is because the very practice of medicine always gets mediated within the social, cultural, and historical context. Not only is the above notion of medicine more humanised, but it also opens up the scope for examining systems of medicine other than biomedicine with equal rigor.

1.6   Medical Care as Provisioning and Culture

The term medical care is most often used to convey those aspects related to provisioning of medical care. This could be due to the quantum of work carried out in the field of provisioning of health care in general and medical care in particular. Here, the major concern is with regard to the inequitable distribution of health services whose reasons are sought within the socio-historic and political context prevalent in societies. This approach implicitly accepts the ability of medicine to be unquestionably beneficial. Then, what is an appropriate term to denote the nature and characteristics of care rendered by a physician to the patient who is unwell? To be more precise, how do we denote those acts happening within the microcosm of an institution, where the act of diagnosis, prognosis, and therapeutics takes place through the engagement of physician and the patient? I would like to consider this also as medical care but for the purpose of distinction it will be henceforth mentioned as the *culture of medical care.* A considerable amount of literature exists on both these aspects of medical care, where the former has been an area of concern predominantly among policy makers whereas the latter has been dealt with extensively by sociologists and medical anthropologists. The latter aspect of medical care also emerged as a *cultural critique* by raising questions about the efficacy of biomedicine with a caution about various iatrogeneses that medicine can induce, resulting in a dependency that at times can be disastrous (Ehrenreich 1978). This difference of opinion has resulted in a kind of non-congruence between the above two perspectives where provisioning recommends for a universal coverage of the dominant system of medical care whilst the latter raises the critical question, do we need to universalise a problematic system of medical care? This incompatibility has led those belonging to the former group to completely reject the latter, as this argument can also be appropriated by conservatives as a justification for cuts in health services (Ehrenreich 1978). Despite this, it is possible that a socialist health policy can be made possible by creating a dialectical understanding of the crisis in medical care by responding to both concerns. This is possible from a *culture of medical care* approach by conceptualising dependency, professionalism, and technology within biomedicine as either due to inadequate provisioning or due to the inherent problems of biomedicine per se, or a combination of both. This in turn can generate notions of rationality in determining methods and systems for effective care, of disciplining people in obtaining and using skills, and of the need to regulate excess belief in medical authority. In other words, there is a scope of questioning the nature of society in which we live and the culture we are constantly engaging with, where medicine is only an extension of the culture we live in and medical care fundamentally becomes a social relationship rather than merely being a commercial or technical one.

1.7 The Sociology of Medical Knowledge

A close examination of the culture of medical care reveals the ways by which the production of medical knowledge happens, the details of which need elaboration. Fleck (1979), known for his book *Genesis and Development of a Scientific Fact*, a pioneering work in the sociology of medical knowledge, set out to show that the knowledge of the natural medical sciences was also a representation, a product of the social (Trenn 1981). This Fleck explains using the concept of *thought style*. He defines thought style as:

> [t]he special ability, be it called basic training, expert knowledge, gift of observation, skill, or what you will, can and must be investigated. It must not be regarded (as happens frequently) as a metaphysical agent, a sacrament which acts absolutely, through its very existence. (Trenn 1981: 254)

For Fleck, the discoveries of scientific facts (medical knowledge) depend not on the discovery of a pre-existing nature, but on the theories we have about that nature. He extends a sociological analysis of science, demonstrating that discovery of scientific facts depends on non-scientific factors such as religious, political, or economic considerations. He furthers the argument by saying that scientific knowledge is collective knowledge, historically located and the product of inter-actions between competing groups with alternative definitions of reality (Fleck 1981[1935]). This he demonstrates by studying syphilis, tracking how an under-standing of it changed through history from a linkage to the position of stars, to a venereal disease because of its reaction to heavy metals, and finally to an aetio-logical notion. In addition, the work on the discovery of the Wasserman reaction— the test for syphilis that was developed in 1906—helped Fleck to advance the argument that progress in medicine is a social and political event, dependent upon thought collectives, rather than a rational scientific event (White 2002). Löwy (1993) demonstrates how the development of the Wassermann reaction emerged as an event that could resolve the four thought styles that were then prevalent about syphilis. Thereafter, a post-Wasserman understanding of syphilis was based on research that was motivated by moral outrage about sexual promiscuity, instigated for political reasons by civil authorities, within the context of nation-state rivalries around biochemical discovery (ibid.). Thus social, political, and moral factors that bind scientists result in a *thought collective* that generates research topics and guides their outcome. Fleck's work was overlooked during his period and only gained acceptance by the 1970s.

Until then, the sociology of medical knowledge did not concern itself with the knowledge claims of biomedicine. Wright and Treacher (1982, cited in White 2002: 15) identify this as being due to four presuppositions. *First*, medicine and medical knowledge were taken for granted by sociologists, which may have resulted in focussing research on achievements of medicine and their institutions as well as on proposed individualistic explanations of social change, i.e. achievements of medi-cine were traced back to great hospitals and great individuals. *Second*, medicine as a part of the natural sciences was granted an epistemologically privileged position, resulting in disease being treated as a natural object and thus preventing its soci-ological inquiry. *Third*, this notion of dominance of the natural sciences made sociologists of medicine tend to consider the social contribution of disease as limited only to epidemiology. *Fourth*, it was thought that for medicine to advance it had to distance itself from the social.

These four claims have been challenged in recent times. The first two were opposed by studies on the sociology of professions in general and the medical profession in particular. Friedson (1970) has extensively studied the sociology of professions, especially the medical profession. He argues that the medical profes-sion dominated the health sector, not because it was the humanitarian scientific elite that it portrays itself to be, but because it was politically well organised. It has a monopoly of practice guaranteed by the state, enjoys autonomy over its own work, and defines for the wider society the issues over which medicine has control. Moreover, medicine's claim to study natural objects has been disputed by the argument that the profession itself can re-define knowledge, thus enhancing power —the power in turn enhancing their knowledge. Lupton (1994) identifies medical profession's monopoly over knowledge that serves to support the professions' powerful position by maintaining patient dependency. Going further, the power of medical practitioners over their work based upon their professional status and autonomy is maintained by their control over medical knowledge. Extending this examination of the power of medicine and medical knowledge, several scholars have studied the medicalisation of everyday life [Illich (1976), Waitzkin (1979), Zola (1972), Crawford 1980)]. Illich and Zola's approach has already been mentioned. Crawford (1980: 368) chooses the word *healthism* to illustrate the act of medicalisation. He defines:

> …healthism as the pre-occupation with personal health as primary—often the primary focus for the definition and achievement of well-being, a goal primarily attained through modification of lifestyles with or without therapeutic help. The aetiology of disease may be seen as complex, but healthism treats individual behaviour, attitudes and emotions as the relevant symptoms needing attention.

By *healthism*, Crawford meant the *normality* of human beings whose violation needs medical attention. In other words, he strongly critiques the biomedical notion of an *ideal, normal* body as healthy, where medicalisation—at least for Crawford— is simply the manifestation of society's notion of *healthism*.

The third claim was nullified by anthropologists like Kleinman, who holds that biomedicine like any other system of medicine is in itself an ethnomedicine. This is based on the view that biomedicine is the *pre-eminent professional ethnomedicine of Western cultures*, as it is based on explanations that reduce pathology to that of universal elementary laws resulting in a problematic medical model of disease (Kleinman 1986). In other words, like any other specialised profession, medicine does not necessarily make sense to those who are not socialised to it.

Fourthly, the contributions of the Foucault-inspired approach are undoubtedly one of the most important contemporary justifications for the recognition of the social or cultural definition of medical phenomena (White 2002). For Foucault, the very seductiveness of modern societies is productive rather than simply confining. The reason for the sustenance of power is simply the fact that it fails to exert its power on the society as a force, rather it diffuses and spreads in the society, produces things, induces pleasure, forms knowledge, and produces discourse. It needs to be considered as a productive network that runs through the whole social body much more than as a negative instance whose function is repression (Lupton 1994: 98–100). In other words, a new way of understanding the *medicalisation* of society was made possible by analysing the very exercise of medical power in terms of local practices, the power of medicine to cure, its ability to predict, and so on. Thus, considering medicine as a *discourse* that produces its own objects helps to open up medical practice to sociological analysis like any other social institution. The orthodox medicalisation critique mentioned elsewhere is similar to this, but Foucault goes further in asserting that there is no such thing as an *authentic* human body that exists outside medical discourse and practice (ibid.). For medical knowledge, Foucault's approach is criticised for his un-sociological treatment of his own subject matter, as it is poorly grounded in the detailed analysis of social organisation of everyday practice. His *discourse* is normally anchored in an adequate representation of the social, but seems to float free of any specific context (ibid. 102–103). Besides, there was not adequate mention of the power of the human body (patient) to resist medical power, thereby nullifying the role of patients in the discourse (ibid.).

Atkinson (1995) considers medical knowledge as produced and reproduced through socially organised practices and transactions by which facts, findings, representations, opinions, and diagnosis occur (ibid.). He categorises these *socially organised practices and transactions* together as *medical work*. This approach preserves the principle of symmetry in order to approach any and all aspects of medical understanding, as was the earlier case with patients and their responses to medicine. In other words, the same logic with which the patient's knowledge, attitude, and practice during illness are examined is also applied to the physician. Thus, it becomes the task of the sociologist and anthropologist to recognise *all* knowledge—scientific, medical, and cultural—that is socially produced within a given setting. This task is strengthened upon close examination of the major actors in the act of medical practice that takes place within the networks of the clinic.

1.8   The Study

This study attempts to interpret discussions about fever in Kerala society among various social groups so as to gain an understanding of its conceptualisation. In addition inquiry into the nature and types of disease—epidemic fevers—will complete the above initiative, as the complexity within the understanding of fever is closely linked to the dominant understanding of those diseases with fever as the major symptom. The media and more importantly, the biomedical system—the dominant medical system and the way it is organised—will all be subjected to rigorous analysis under fever treatment, as their functioning can influence the dominant understanding. Understanding the interrelationship between the notions of fevers and the nature and characteristics of biomedicine, as well as the extent of medicalisation and risk perceived by society, will promote an understanding of the response of people towards the illness. This is to reassert the fact that any kind of analysis in isolation will be inadequate to demonstrate the problem completely.

Fever is conceptualised as a discourse in Kerala society that has varied meanings depending on the context, wherein fever care is comprised of (1) provisioning, a function of the nature of organisation of medical care, and (2) the culture of fever care, a function of the biomedical understanding and interpretation of fevers. This calls for an analysis that situates provisioning largely as a question of government policy as well as people's access to services, while the culture of fever care is seen as what ought to be fever care (practice of medicine) and its contribution to medical knowledge. With this, the broad objective of the study was to explore how fever patients are rendered care by allopathic hospitals in the present scenario, giving due consideration to the sociocultural context of the patients and doctors as well as the prevalent discourse about fevers in the society.

Thus, the present book traces the understanding of fever by the lay public and examines it against the biomedical interpretation of fevers. This is situated within the larger context of the state of Kerala, known for its better health status, greater access to health services, and for the contemporary reality of a threat of fever epidemics in the population. It is in this context that the establishment of fever clinics is examined along with a close look at the functioning of the clinic in terms of the procedures of diagnosis, prognosis, and treatment within the facility. Finally, the diverse interpretation of fevers by the community in contemporary times unravels the extent to which medicalisation and risk interfere with the under-standing of a minor illness like fever. Additionally, treatment-seeking behaviour of those affected demonstrates how risk perception and medicalisation become an opportunity for commercialisation even with a minor illness like fever. Finally, a microanalysis within the ethnography of a clinic reveals how social context inter-feres with the core of medical practice and demonstrates how medicine, while aspiring to become more 'scientific', transforms itself to laboratory medicine, thus becoming a vehicle to the new field of medical care— preventive diagnostics. The doctor–patient interaction and its meaning are analysed and interpreted using narrative analysis.

1.9 The Setting

The present section covers the settings of the study, as making explicit the setting of the field is the only way by which credibility of an anthropological study can be achieved (Sanjek 1990). The setting described here will have two sub-sections: first, the sociocultural and development context of Kerala along with a morbidity and health care scenario, and second, a detailed description of the four hospitals in which the ethnography of fever care was carried out.

1.9.1 Social Development in Kerala

Kerala state in India is known for its development despite its low per-capita income, with many of its social indicators comparable to that of developed countries (Franke and Chasin 1991; Tharamangalam 1998). These include improvements in educa-tion, as reflected in a higher literacy rate, and health indicators like low infant mortality rate, low birth rate, and significantly good life expectancy (ibid.). Another notable feature within Kerala is the fact that the achievements are distributed more or less equally across rural and urban areas and between the male and female population, and that inequality is comparatively less between classes (Tharamangalam 1998). In other words, the majority of Kerala's families are in middle-income groups, with fewer families among the extreme poor as compared to other Indian states, which implies that income disparity is less severe than in other states (Pillai et al. 2003). The above state of development, also known as the Kerala model of development, is attributed to historical movements and a people's struggle that led to land reforms and social reform movements, as well as to Kerala's unique ecological and geographical factors (Tharamangalam 1998; Franke and Chasin 1991). These culminated in increased political consciousness, which resulted in the people's demand for basic facilities like education, health, and food as an inherent right of their citizenship. The following section will be confined to the debates surrounding the nature and characteristics of the health of the people and health services prevalent in the state.

1.9.2 Kerala's Morbidity and Health Care Scenario

The disease pattern during the 1990s remained more or less similar to that of the 1980s. An increase occurred in non-communicable disease load, indicating that epidemiological transition is taking place in the state. Detailed analysis on the pattern of communicable diseases and fevers in particular help us to understand the situation better. There has been a decline in waterborne diseases, especially diarrhoea, which is attributed to improved sanitation and water supply (Kunjhikannan and Aravindan 2000). The prevalence of measles, mumps, tetanus, and filariasis is less than 0.5 per 1000 population. TB prevalence is a bit high, at around 1.32 per 1000, whereas that of fevers is 67.95 per 1000 (Kunjhikannan and Aravindan 2000). The category of 'fevers' here includes diseases like viral fevers, upper and lower respiratory tract infections, simple cough, and runny nose, which are quite common. At any one time, 6.7–7.9 % of the state's population suffers from these illnesses. This was estimated based on the community survey conducted over a two-week period that included questions on the symptoms of fever. This becomes convincing when one looks at the data on outpatient attendance of primary health centres (PHCs), where nearly 30–40 % of all outpatient attendance in PHCs and other peripheral institutions is solely due to fevers and/or respiratory infections (Kunjhikannan and Aravindan 2000). The recent National Sample Survey Office (NSSO) 71st round on morbidity also identifies fevers as a major category among both outpatient illnesses and hospitalisation cases. Despite the fact that fevers are the most prevalent illness in the state, they have not been adequately studied. The reason for this could probably be the fact that fevers have been known since antiquity and are considered a symptom by the public, and so they carry a notion of being a common, natural problem. There also exist notions among doctors and health planners that fevers are over-reported due to the unique feature that they can be a symptom for a range of diseases, and therefore many other diseases may also get reported as fevers. Non-communicable diseases or diseases of affluence are also on the rise in Kerala, a consistent feature revealed by the studies of Panicker and Soman (1984), Kannan et al. (1991), and later by Kunjhikannan and Aravindan (2000) and recent surveys (Aravindan 2006; NSSO 71st round). Though diseases due to poverty have been reduced over the period, there has been a resurgence of new epidemics in the state during the 1990s. Thus the state is said to face a dual crisis, both of diseases of poverty and diseases of affluence, giving rise to questions on whether an epidemiological transition is really happening (Panicker 1999).

One factor that scholars have identified as contributing to the development of health of the people is demographic transition (Ratcliffe 1978). This is broadened to health transition, which encompasses demographic, epidemiological, and health care transition. The major characteristics of current demographic transition are low mortality and low fertility with significantly lower infant mortality and greater life expectancy. The above demographic transition is offered as an explanation for the decrease in communicable diseases and rise in non-communicable diseases, a feature of epidemiological transition (Panicker 1999). Here, the shift in age struc-ture of the morbid population is seen also as an outcome of the above demographic transition. From an epidemiological point of view, it was found that after the 1970s a tremendous improvement took place in the health indicators of the state. A paradox of these indicators in Kerala is that despite the increase in morbidity rate, mortality rate has been very low. This is attributed to the greater coverage of the health services system in the state and also to the higher health consciousness of the people (Panicker and Soman 1984; Kannan et al. 1991, Kunjhikannan and Aravindan 2000). The higher health consciousness is also interpreted as due to a perception factor that has been the feature of societies where access to health services is greater (Murray and Chen 1992). In other words, the higher health consciousness of people is conceived as an individualistic characteristic, namely perceived morbidity. This is reasserted when some scholars argue that perceived morbidity for Kerala is very high (Kunjhikannan and Aravindan 2000). It is worth mentioning at this juncture that when examined in the social context, the perception factor appears to be more an outcome of a medicalised society, one of the features of modern society.

1.9.3   The Hospital Setting

The description of the four hospitals at this juncture is inevitable, since making the settings of the field explicit is necessary in order to better interpret the context. A general description on the commonalties found in all hospitals will be attempted here and a detailed description will follow. It is well known that hospitals in general perform a range of functions of which those related to fever care alone will be focussed on, as the study is confined only to that aspect. Broadly, the procedures involved in all these hospitals can be divided into two, viz. administrative function and medical function. The former is comprised of the processes of registration leading to the making of a case record, which remain as the identity of those who seek care and later the cost of the care usually collected as cash or otherwise. The remaining function of medical care comprises a diagnosis accomplished through laboratory investigations, physical examination, history taking, and so on, along with a prognosis and therapeutics, together treated as medical work. This will be the major focus here because the latter procedures are considered the core of medical practice where the objectification of lay categories happens and thereby contributes to medical knowledge. Thus, the study will be more concerned with the latter aspect of the process of diagnosis and therapeutic decision-making. It should be noted that the names given for the hospitals and the patients in this book are purposefully changed to ensure anonymity and confidentiality of the information.

1.10   Theoretical Framework

As mentioned earlier the study traverses through diverse perspectives to accomplish its objectives. It becomes difficult to underpin one single framework throughout the work, as different perspectives are used to make sense of each area of inquiry. This might appear as a shortcoming but also is a strength, as the study of an illness only becomes meaningful when diverse dimensions of the same event are captured through thick descriptions. Thus, talk about fever that involves multiple interpretations of the same event and during different phases of life, along with the government response to a crisis through the establishment of a fever clinic are interpreted using discourse analysis. Further, the risk perception about an epidemic and the nature and characteristics of a medicalised society are revealed using ethnography. Additionally, the culture of fever care is captured using ethnomethodology inspired by the science studies framework, and finally, the doctor–patient interaction is interpreted through narrative analysis.

In order to accomplish the above, the study was carried out broadly at four levels. First, the discourses on fever at various levels were examined. This was based on the history of Western medicine in general and fevers in particular by tracing the evolution of Western medicine in the West, India, and more importantly, in the state of Kerala. Discourses around fever among the medical fraternity and health professionals were predominantly based on archival reports and documents on fever brought out during the epidemic that were collected from government institutions and other libraries. Gaining a sense of how fever is understood by public health officials was based mostly on government documents, official statistics, minutes of government level meetings, and so on. This was supplemented with semi-structured personal interviews with government officials about fevers and the state-level initiatives to control the problem. Additionally, newspaper reports on fever, fever clinics, and fever deaths were an excellent source through which to understand the discourse among the lay public as well as in the media, as scholars have acknowledged the vibrant role of the newspaper in Kerala society (Jeffrey 1997). Additionally, focus group discussions at different stages with various groups helped to illuminate people's perspective on fevers and the difficulties faced in experiencing them. As the context of the establishment of a fever clinic in May 2004 was one of the focuses of the study, minutes of all intersectoral and health official meetings held during 2002–2004 in the directorate of health services were reviewed. The notion of fevers among government officials and the discussions that took place as part of the establishment of fever clinics were traced based on government documents, minutes of government-level meetings held among different groups, and other relevant reports from the four study hospitals.

Second, an interpretation of fevers among those affected was carried out by examining the patterns of distress, perceived causes, and patterns of help-seeking behaviour. This was superimposed on the general health-seeking pattern among people and the nature of health care institutions, their mandates, and their interpretations of fever. Further, within a health policy framework, the study examined the population characteristics and the burden created by a minor illness while receiving treatment in a public and private setting and their implications for the provisioning of medical care in general. 'Interview Schedule' was used as a tool to capture data on various interpretations of fever among those affected, covering information on patients' access and utilisation of the services and their perception of fever at various instances, its perceived cause, treatment, and cure, and relevant socio-economic, political, cultural, and ecological contexts. Supplementing this were in-depth interviews of a few patients on specific issues, as well as of the doctors on their day-to-day work, government-level interventions to control the epidemic, and other relevant issues.

The third aspect of the study, the culture of fever care, was based on the study of hospital as a microcosm where each hospital is treated as a unit with special reference to fever care. Diverse factors can influence the functioning of a hospital depending on the sector (public or private) as well as the level to which each hospital belongs. However, commonalties exist in terms of the procedures involved and the nature of the outcomes (i.e. the medical practice), as these derive from a common origin in terms of the system of medicine practised, which is biomedicine. These differences and commonalties can be revealed only through the procedures involved in fever care, which has been the concern of the researcher. This calls for a detailed ethnography of the hospital, covering the procedures (events), the actors and artefacts involved, and the dynamic interaction of all these together constituting medical work. The major tool used in this was passive participant observation. This method can be traced to (Spradley 1980: 58–60), who argues that participant observation as a method itself can consist of different kinds depending on the degree of participation (passive, moderate, active, complete) in the social situation. He elaborates that passive participation is a situation where the researcher finds an observation post, from where he finds and records what is going on, taking the role of a bystander or spectator. This was supplemented by several interviews (mostly informal) as part of clarifications from the doctors, patients, and other actors involved in the events, which also help in triangulation of the information generated.

The fourth aspect involves the doctors and patients; their interactions were observed and recorded, and their conversations were treated as text and subjected to narrative analysis (Czarniawska 2004). Here, the process of clinical decision-making as well as the response of the patient was examined within the context, and also in terms of its influence on the outcome of fever care. Moreover, the doctor–

patient interaction during the clinical encounter was observed for a considerable number of cases, giving due consideration to the context of the interactions.

1.11 Secondary-Level Hospitals: The District Hospital and the Immanuel Hospital

The basic infrastructure facilities available for the four hospitals selected are elaborated upon here for a better understanding of the features of the hospital. Both the secondary hospitals (district and Immanuel) have bed strength of more than 300 —for the district hospital it is around 500. Both have emergency facilities and laboratory facilities capable of doing routine biochemical tests. In addition, a public health laboratory is attached to the district hospital where facilities for immunoglobulin and enzyme-linked immunosorbent assay (ELISA) tests for dengue, leptospirosis, AIDS, etc., are available; this feature is absent in the case of the Immanuel hospital. In both hospitals, there are specialisations for general medicine, paediatrics, ENT, ophthalmology, orthopaedic, skin and venereal diseases, and others. The Immanuel hospital is especially known for its specialisation in the field of ophthalmology and cardiology. Generally, both these hospitals do not depend on laboratories other than their own for rendering fever care. In the Immanuel hospital three general physicians were present and consulting on a daily basis, whereas in the district hospital three physicians and three house surgeons worked together, each making a pair during daily rounding with the patients depending on their allotted days.

1.12 Public Hospital at the Primary Level: Community Health Centre

The hospital at the primary level selected from the government sector was a recently upgraded community health centre (CHC), with 16 beds available for inpatients; the centre also implements and monitors public health activities (communicable disease control, health education, etc.) in its catchment area. As this hospital is responsible for community-level control programmes for TB, malaria, filariasis, and blindness, the laboratory only has the facilities to perform sputum tests for TB, blood smear tests for malaria and filariasis, and urine tests for diabetes and eye testing. This created a situation in which physicians are forced to ask their patients to get simple lab tests (routine biochemical tests e.g. blood and urine) from private laboratories located on the hospital premises. This results in additional burden for the majority of poor patients coming to this public sector hospital for treatment.

1.13   Sivani Hospital

Sivani hospital, the private hospital at the primary level, is functioning in a building that was previously a house and is now modified into a hospital, which itself gives a different outlook to the whole institution. The hospital is very old and run by a single, well-liked doctor, around 60 years old, who started his practice during the 1970s with a good reputation of being simple and effective in medical care. There are 18 beds, as well as facilities for basic laboratory tests, a dressing room for wounds, a pharmacy, and so on. This was the only hospital among the four where the doctor regularly used a thermometer to record temperatures for patients presenting with complaints of fever. In this hospital the doctor generally treats a range of minor illnesses, and in the event of serious illness or those that fail to respond to his treatment, he refers cases to any other hospital in consultation with the patient. Additionally, if required, for some patients he also prescribes certain laboratory tests to be carried out at other private laboratories.

1.14   Commonalties and Differences in Hospital Procedures

In all of the four hospitals, registration of the patient is the first step for any patient coming to the doctor for consultation. The registration fee was Re. 1 in the CHC and Rs. 2 for the district hospital, whereas it was Rs. 65 for Immanuel Hospital and Rs. 20–30 for Sivani hospital, decided by the physician depending on the nature of the illness and the patient's socio-economic status.

In the Immanuel hospital, Rs. 50 of the total fee of Rs. 65 is the doctor's consultation fee for a period of one month, which means that the patient can consult the respective doctor any number of times during this period. The remaining Rs. 15 covers the registration fees of the hospital. It is worth mentioning here that this could be a mechanism of marketing strategy that increases dependence on medical care, as the doctor's fee covers consultation for any diseases that may arise over the one-month period. Subsequent to the registration process, a case record is made in which the name, age, sex, address of the patient, and the name of the doctor to be consulted are also depicted. This is carried out by the clerical staff of the hospital, thereby transforming the identity of a person to that of a patient. Then the patient waits to consult with a physician in the space allotted within the hospital outside the consulting room. This space and the facilities provided in the waiting room (area) vary widely among public and private hospitals.

In the public sector (the district hospital and the CHC), the facility for sitting is often inadequate, resulting in a majority of the patients standing for long hours before consultation. Eventually, according to the order of registration, patients enter the consulting room when called by a hospital attendant in both of the hospitals. In the case of the private hospitals (Immanuel and Sivani), physicians' attendants, specific for each physician, allow the patients to enter the consultation room one-by-one based on the order of registration.

The consulting rooms of the two secondary hospitals (the district hospital and Immanuel hospital) are set up similarly. A table is placed at the centre of the room, around which chairs and stools are arranged in such a manner that one chair and one stool form a pair, making two consultations possible at a time whenever two physicians are available. In the primary hospitals (the CHC and Sivani hospital), the arrangement was set up for only one physician at a time. On the table at all of the hospitals were kept the instruments for checking blood pressure, a set of papers (forms) for prescribing lab tests, and a set of sample medicines, mostly given by medical representatives. Additionally, in the private hospitals instruments like tongue depressors immersed in a chemical solution were also kept on the table. A thermometer immersed in a solution was kept only in the Sivani hospital. It should be noted that there is a huge difference in the quality of facilities available in the public and private hospitals, though there is not much difference in the quantity of articles. This becomes obvious upon learning that the entire consultation and waiting room areas of the district hospital occupy an amount of space equal to that of the Immanuel hospital consulting room alone. In the former, the consulting room and the waiting room are divided only by a cloth screen with iron frame, whereas for the latter, they consist of two rooms with separate entrances. Moreover, in both of the private hospitals, there is an examination table arranged inside the consulting room separated by a screen and a curtain, which in the public hospitals is a stretcher kept at the corner of the room that is occasionally used for physical examination.

The procedures for consultation are such that the doctor and patient interact for the first time, and based on the patient's explanation, the doctor records the details of the illness in a particular format in the case record. Subsequently, the patient is subjected to physical examination and laboratory investigations as the case demands, and thereafter is asked to meet with the doctor for the results. The doctor may then prescribe medicines for a short period and ask the patient to come for a follow-up if required. The extent of physical examinations carried out, laboratory investigations prescribed, and prescription patterns all depend on each case that calls for an analysis, taking into consideration the context as it is influenced by a range of factors. The hospital setting discussed above will help to create an understanding of the medical care scenario prevalent in the community and will therefore help to illustrate the context of fever care.

1.15   'Being a Participant Observer'

Two scenarios were prevalent with certain commonalities, since the type of patients traced was confined to that of fever patients. Their status as patients within the society is acceptable and carries the least stigma, generally being treated as having a 'normal' illness, at least in the initial stages. The first scenario was of the private hospitals, where there were only a few patients (8–10 patients per doctor per day) and where privacy and confidentiality are valued more by the administration and the doctor, mainly due to a lower patient load. Here, before the patients entered the doctor's consultation room, they were approached about participating in the study, offered an explanation, and based on prior permission from the hospital and the consulting physician, I then essentially assumed the role of a bystander to the patient during consultation. This was possible because more than one person was allowed to be in the room with the patient during consultation, along with the nursing staff and assistants who all witness the doctor–patient interaction.

The second scenario was that of the public sector hospitals, where the number of patients are large (150–200 patients per doctor per day). Here, the very concept of privacy and confidentiality in medical practice itself are at stake, as those patients who are waiting for consultation can clearly see and hear what each patient and doctor communicates. In this scenario, I was also sitting with the doctor throughout the sessions, and observed and documented those interactions that I felt relevant and important to capture. Here, it is important to gauge ethics according to context. I recall Riessman's (2005) description of her experience with ethical standards while conducting research in southern Indian medical settings, where she argues that privacy, confidentiality, and informed consent within social research must be engaged in differently in settings where these are not even followed in medical practice. While performing social inquiry into those medical practices, one needs to develop what Riessman calls 'ethics-in-context', which according to her is that which 'provides room for particularities that unfold during fieldwork' (ibid.; 487). This again underscores the importance of context, not only in narrative production but also in formulating one's ethical standpoint.

References

Ananth, Mahesh. (2008). *In defense of an evolutionary concept of health: Nature, norms and human biology*. United Kingdom: Ashgate.

Aravindan, K. P. (2006). *Kerala padanam, keralam engane Jeevikkunnu? Keralalm engane chinthikkunnu?(Malayalam): A Study on Kerala, How Kerala lives? How Kerala thinks?*. Kozhikode, Kerala. Kerala Sastra Sahitya Parishad.

Armstrong, D. (1995). The rise of surveillance medicine. *Sociology of Health & Illness, 17*(3), 393–404.

Atkinson, Paul. (1995). *Medical talk and medical work: The liturgy of the clinic*. London: Sage Publications.

Boorse, C. (1976). On the distinction between disease and illness. *Philosophy & Public Affairs, 5*(1), 49–68.

Brown, M. W. (1985). On defining 'disease'. *The Journal of Medicine and Philosophy, 10*, 311–328.

Bury, M. (1998). Postmodernity and Health. In Graham Scambler & Paul Higgs (Eds.), *Modernity medicine and health, medical sociology towards 2000* (pp. 1–28). London and New York: Routledge.

Canguilhem, G. (1991). *On the normal and the pathological*. New York: Zone Books.

Cartwright, F. F. (1977). *A social history of medicine*. London: Longman.

Crawford, R. (1980). Healthism and medicalisation of everyday life. *International Journal of Health Services, 10*(3), 365–388.

Czarniawska, B. (2004). *Narratives in social science research*. London: Sage.

Ehrenreich, J. (1978). Introduction. In J. Ehrenreich (Ed.), *The cultural crisis of modern medicine* (pp. 1–35). New York: Monthly Review Press.

Engel, G. L. (1977). The need for a new medical model: a challenge for biomedicine. *Science, 196* (4286), 129–136.

Engelhardt, T., Jr. (1976). Ideology and etiology, *The Journal of Medicine and Philosophy, 1*, 3, 256–268.

Fleck, L. (1979). *Genesis and development of a scientific fact*. Chicago: University of Chicago Press.

Fleck, L. (1981[1935]). On the question of the foundation of medical knowledge. *Journal of Medicine and Philosophy, 6*(3), 237–56.

Foucault, M. (1975). *The birth of the clinic: Archaeology of medical perception*. New York and London: Vintage Books.

Franke, R., & Chasin, B. (1991). Kerala State, India: Radical reform as development. *Monthly Review, 42*(8), 1–23.

Friedson, E. (1970). *The professions of medicine: A study of the sociology of applied knowledge*. Dodd, New York: Mead.

Gallagher, E. R. (1976). Lines of Reconstruction and Extension in the Parsonian Sociology of Illness. *Social Science and Medicine*, 10, 207–218.

George, M. (2014a). Book review: Mahesh Ananth (2008) In defense of an evolutionary concept of health: Nature, norms and human biology. *Medicine Studies: An International Journal of History, Philosophy, and Ethics of Medicine and Allied Sciences, 4*(4), 113–117.

Gerhardt, U. (1987). Parsons' role theory and health interaction. In G. Scambler (Ed.), *Sociological theory and medical sociology*. London: Routledge.

Good, B. J. (1994). *Medicine, rationality and experience, an anthropological experience*. Cambridge: Cambridge University Press.

Illich, I. (1976). *Medical nemesis: The expropriation of medical knowledge*. Calcutta: Calder and Boyars.

Jeffrey, R. (1997) Malayalam: 'The day–to–day Social Life of the People…', *Economic and Political Weekly*, January 4–11, 32, 1 & 2, 18–21.

Kannan, K. P., Thankappan, K. R., Ramankutty, V., & Aravindan, K. P. (1991). *Health and development in Rural Kerala*. Thiruvananthapuram, Kerala: Kerala Sastra Sahithya Parishad.

Kasl, S. V., & Cobb, S. (1966). Health behaviour, illness behaviour, and sick role behaviour. *Archives of Environmental Health, 12*, 246–266.

King, L. S. (1982). *Medical thinking. A historical preface*. Princeton, New Jersey: Princeton University Press.

Kleinman, A. (1980). *Patients and healers in the context of culture. An exploration of the borderland between anthropology, medicine and psychiatry*. Berkeley: University of California Press.

Kleinman, A. (1986). Concepts and a model for the comparison of medical systems as cultural systems. In C. Currer & M. Stacey (Eds.), *Concepts of health, illness and disease* (pp. 29–47). Oxford: Berg Publications Ltd.

Kleinman, A., Eisenberg, L., & Good, B. (1978). Culture, illness and care, clinical lessons form anthropologic and cross-cultural research. *Annals of Internal Medicine, 88*, 251–258.

Kraupl Taylor, F. (1980). The concept of disease. *Psychological Medicine, 10*, 419–424.

Kunjhikannan, T. P., & Aravindan, K. P. (2000). *Changes in health transition in Kerala, 1987–1997*. Thiruvananthapuram: Kerala Research Programme on Local Level Development, Centre for Development Studies.

Latour and Woolgar. (1986). *The laboratory life: The construction of scientific facts*. Princeton, New Jersey: Princeton University Press.

Löwy, I. (1993). Testing for a sexually transmissible disease 1907–1970: The history of the wassermann reaction. In V. Berridge & P. Strong (eds.), *Aids, and contemporary history* (pp. 74–92). Cambridge: Cambridge University press.

Lupton, D. (1994). *Medicine as culture: Illness, disease and the body in the western societies.* London: Sage.

Mechanic, D. (1969). Illness and cure. In J. Kosa, et al. (Eds.), *Poverty and health—a sociological analysis.* London: Harvard University.

Munson, R. (1981). Why medicine cannot be a science. *The Journal of Medicine and Philosophy, 6*, 183–208.

Murray, C. J., & Chen, L. (1992). Understanding morbidity change. *Population and Development Review, 48*, 481–503.

Navarro, V. (1975). The political economy of medical care, an explanation of the compositions, nature and functions of the present health sector of The United States. *International Journal of Health Services, 5*(1), 65–94.

Navarro, V. (1986). *Crisis, health, and medicine, a social critique.* New York: Tavistock Publications.

NSSO *Key Indicators of Social Consumption in India: Health*, (NSSO 71st Round, January–June 2014); 2015: A8.

Panicker, P.G.K. (1999) *Health transition in Kerala.* Discussion Paper No. 10, Thiruvananthapuram, Kerala: Kerala Research Programme on Local Level Development, Centre For Development Studies.

Panicker, P. G. K., & Soman, C. R. (1984). *Health status of Kerala: The paradox of economic backwardness and health development.* Thiruvananthapuram, Kerala: Centre for Development Studies.

Parsons, T. (1951). *The social system.* London: Routledge and Kegan Paul.

Pellegrino, E. D., & Thomasma, D. (1981) *A philosophical basis of medical practice, toward a philosophy and ethic of the healing professions*, New York and Oxford: Oxford University Press.

Pillai, R. K., Williams, S. V., Glick, H. A., et al. (2003). Factors affecting decisions to seek treatment for sick children in Kerala. *India, Social Science and Medicine, 57*, 783–790.

Ratcliffe, J. (1978). Social justice and the demographic transition: Lessons from India's Kerala State. *International Journal of Health Services, 8*(1), 123–144.

Reiser, J. S. (1978). *Medicine and the reign of technology.* Cambridge, United Kingdom: Cambridge University Press.

Reissman, C. K. (2005) Exporting ethics: A narrative about narrative research in south India. *Health: An Interdisciplinary Journal for the Social Study of Health, Illness and Medicine, 9*(4), 473–490.

Rosenberg, C. E. (1989). Disease in history: Frames and framers. *The Milbank Quarterly, 67*(1), 1–15.

Rosenberg, C. (2002). The tyranny of diagnosis, specific entities and individual experience. *The Millbank Quarterly, 80*(2), 237–60.

Sanjek, R. (1990) On ethnographic validity. In R. Sanjek (ed.), *Fieldnotes, the makings of anthropology.* Ithaca and London: Cornell University Press.

Spradley, J. P. (1980). *Participant observation.* Australia and United Kingdom: Wadsworth, Thomson Learning.

Suchman, E. A. (1963). *Sociology and the field of public health.* New York: Russell Sage Foundation.

Sujatha, V. (2014) *Sociology of health and medicine: New perspectives.* Oxford: Oxford University Press.

Tharamangalam, J. (1998). The perils of social development without economic growth: The development debacle of Kerala, India. *Bulletin of Concerned Asian Scholars, 30*(1), 23–34.

Trenn, T. J. (1981). Ludwick Fleck's 'on the question of the foundation of medical knowledge'. *Journal of Medicine and Philosophy, 6*, 237–256.

Turner, B. S. (2000). The history of the changing concepts of health and illness: Outline of a general model of illness categories. In G. Albrecht, R. Fitzpatrick, & S. Schrimshaw (Eds.), *Handbook of social studies in health and medicine*. London: Sage.

Waitzkin, H. (1979). Medicine, superstructure and micropolitics. *Social Science and Medicine, 13A*, 601–619.

White, K. (2002). *An introduction to the sociology of health and illness*. London: Sage.

Wulff, H. R. (1990). Function and value of medical knowledge in modern diseases. In H. A. Ten Have, G. K. Kimsam, & S. F. Spicher (Eds.), *The growth of medical knowledge*. London: Kluwer Academic Publishers.

Wright, P., & Treacher, A. (1982) (eds) *The problem of medical knowledge: Examining social construction of medicine*. Edinburgh: Edinburgh University Press.

Young, A. (1981). The creation of medical knowledge. *Some Problems in Interpretation, Social Science and Medicine, 15B*, 376–386.

Young, Allan. (1982). The anthropologies of illness and sickness. *Annual Review of Anthropology, 11*, 257–85.

Zola, I. K. (1972). Medicine as an institution of social control. *Sociological Review, 20*, 487–503.

Chapter 2
Historical Discourses on Fevers

Abstract Fevers have been prevalent in every society since early times, and hence the history of fevers, to a certain extent, is also the history of medicine. As it is obvious that fevers are not a homogeneous category, their classification and distinction during different periods can explain the discourse on fevers during those times. The present chapter attempts to trace the history of fevers, their prevalent types, and the theories and the treatment followed in Western society since the sixteenth century, which is used as a pretext to understanding the Indian experience of fevers since the nineteenth century. This was the context for analysing the history of fever care in the state of Kerala during the 1990s when the 'epidemics' of fever struck the state. This historical inquiry also demonstrates the history of medical care and public health in the Indian subcontinent, especially in the state of Kerala. The history of public health and medical care reveals the distinction in approaches between the two, and the tension in terms of their interaction and areas of operation attains greater significance even in the current context when there is a blurring of boundaries of these two related disciplines. Further, the international influences in public health interventions were also significant then, and remain so even today.

Keywords History of fevers · Epidemics · Public health in Travancore · Medical cosmology fevers in India

2.1 Introduction

The present chapter is an attempt to trace the history of fevers, their prevalent types, the theories about them, and the therapies used to treat them. As fevers were prevalent in every society since early times, the history of fevers to a certain extent is also the history of medicine. However, it is obvious that 'fever' is not a homogeneous category. The classification and distinction of fevers during different periods can explain the discourse on fevers in those times. Thus, in this chapter, the history of fevers in Western society since the sixteenth century will be examined as a pretext to understanding the Indian experience of fevers since the nineteenth

© Springer Science+Business Media Singapore 2017   29
M. George, *Institutionalizing Illness Narratives*,
DOI 10.1007/978-981-10-1905-0_2

century. This will be the context for analysing the history of fever care in the state of Kerala during 1990s when the 'epidemics' of fever struck the state. It is in this milieu that the discourse on fevers in Kerala and the context of establishing fever clinics in the state will be investigated in the next chapter. Bynum and Nutton (1981) cautions that the study of fevers should be limited to inquiry within a researcher's specific purpose, as the study area involves a complex variety of complementary techniques and sources and there is a limit to one's scholarly armour. Historical analyses of fevers envisage not only the forms of response to fever but also the medical personnel's understanding of disease in general. As Pickstone (1992: 128) in his discussion on 'fever' argues:

> ... the changes in ideas about epidemics need to be understood in terms of political theory and medical theory and that these can be fully understood via an historical sociology of knowledge which roots ideas in changing social structures.

2.2 Early History of Fevers in the West

Fevers were identified in the Hippocratic writing as 'acute', with seasonal onset and durations of twenty-one days consisting of three periods of seven days duration; they were also associated with bile during that period (Smith 1981). The importance of bile could possibly have been due to the then-prevalent *humoral theory*, where bile was one of the humours. Additionally, a high fever was treated as dangerous; cessation of fever usually indicated progress towards recovery (ibid.). Fevers were given different names, and often also treated as the primary symptom for certain diseases. Treatments generally included nursing care followed by purgation and nourishment at proper times (ibid.). A special warning to the physician during that period remains relevant even now: 'Do not, if you are the physician, treat wrongly for fear of turning the fever into another worse disease' (ibid: 10). In other words, the role of the physician in the case of fever was more of care than of cure, as fever was seen as the body's means of regaining balance. Later, Galen's fever theory— similar to his general theory of disease[1] and treatment, which relied more on explanation and was unsupported by proof—was accepted as the most valid basis of practice until the twelfth century (Bynum and Nutton 1981: viii, Cartwright 1977). During the second half of the sixteenth century, the Paracelsians contradicted the Galenists, Arabists, and Aristotelians, but were also the forerunners in many subsequent approaches, not only in their contributions to the understanding of fever, but also to medicine as a whole (ibid.).

---

[1]The theory of diseases proposed by Galen combined the *humoral* theory of the Greeks and the Graeco-Roman theory of the *pneuma*. The former consider blood, phlegm, yellow bile, and black bile as the four humours, whose imbalance can lead to disease, and for the latter, *pneuma* is a vital principle carried by the nerves wherein the *origin* of the disease is considered as supernatural with a natural *cause*. For more details, see Cartwright (1977).

Sixteenth-century fever theory was important mainly on two grounds. First, the Paracelsian theory of disease, which identifies pathologic poisons and predisposition as causative factors for any disease, and second, the contribution of Michael Servetus (1553) on the theory of pulmonary circulation of blood, which contradicted Galen's ebb-and-flow movement (Cartwright 1977: 17). Consequently, it was generally agreed upon by the sixteenth century that the nature of fever lay in the 'heat contrary to nature' or had something to do with the heat experienced by the patient (Lonie 1981: 20). In other words, the major focus during this period was on the definition of fever with respect to its well-accepted quality, 'heat', where two types that were opposed to each other were identified, viz. febrile and innate heats.[2] The culmination of the idea of circulation of blood as well as the heat aspect of fever becomes obvious from Avicenna's definition:

> Fever is extraneous heat, kindled in the heart, from which it is diffused to the whole body through the arteries and veins, by means of the spirit and blood, reaching a heat in the body itself which is sufficient to injure the natural functions. (ibid. 21)

Averroes, following Galen, later commented: 'Fever occurs through the conversion of innate heat to the fiery'. He gave an alternate formulation that fever was not merely an extraneous heat but a unity composed of natural and extraneous heat. It is in fact these disparities that set the terms for all subsequent discussions on the relationship between preternatural heat and natural heat (ibid.). In both of these explanations, it should be noted that the two important features during this period were (1) the understanding that heat produces fever and not the other way round, and (2) the centrality of the heart in the production of heat.

2.3   Classification of Fevers

During this period, many tried to explain the nature of fevers in terms of the nature of heat produced but did not succeed. However, based on the substances involved in the production of heat, three[3] genera of fever, *ephemeral, putrid or humoral* and *hectic*, were identified (ibid.). Another form of distinguishing fevers was based on its frequency of presentation, one such being the intermittent fevers. Here, the distinction was based on the observation that there was a precise regularity or intermittency that was independent of age, constitution, diet, and all other variables

---

[2]The terms febrile, preternatural, unnatural, and extraneous heat were used interchangeably and are seen as in opposition to natural or animal heat. Also, one should recall that heat was regarded as a substance, capable of division into different genera and species. This view followed naturally from a cosmology that regarded heat or the hot as one of the four elements of which all things, both animate and inanimate, are composed, and where the three substances of spirits, humours, and flesh jointly compose the substance of innate heat. For details, see Lonie (1981).

[3]Since three substances (spirits, humours, and flesh) jointly compose the substance of innate heat, they respectively produce three genera of fever: ephemeral, putrid, or humoral and hectic.

(ibid.). In other words, the shift in the attempt to understand fever based on its cause (heat) to that based on effect (presentation) has to be seen as a major shift towards what is possible. This is evident from Fernel, whose fever theory later led to an explicit connection with anatomy. He states 'the *contenta* of the body (spirits, humours and excrements) were never the subject of disease, but only its causes: diseases themselves were to be located in the parts of the body, and symptoms in the functions' (cf. ibid. 32). Later, introducing the concept of combustion as an analogy to explain elevated body temperature, scholars attacked the theory that fevers are caused due to putrefaction (imbalance) of humours. With 'heat' identified as the main cause of fever, it was thought that burning (of something) produced the heat, and since putrefaction is related to death as a feature of a cold body, it was ruled out (ibid.). Thus, the feature of fever theory during that period according to Lonie (1981: 41) was that:

> ... the febrile heat is not specifically different from natural heat, but is an effect of the accelerated motion of the heart and arteries, this motion being provoked by a variety of causes, and its purpose being to separate and expel noxious substances from the blood.

Thus, a close examination of the sixteenth-century understanding of fever helps to identify three different features. First, a distinction between febrile and natural heat as the basis for explanation was a common feature throughout the century, though the mechanisms and purposes behind these forms of heat vary. Second, prior to Harvey who propounded his theory of circulation of blood and its relation to the heart one can find mention about the heart and circulation of blood in most of the theories on fever. Lastly, but more importantly, as Lonie (1981: 43) puts it: 'febrile heat was a substantial entity and a causal agent, not the consequence of physiological changes'.

2.4 Fevers During the Sixteenth and Seventeenth Centuries: Descriptive to Problematic

The topic of fever during the seventeenth century was more of a description of what was happening based on experience than of explaining its characteristics. In other words, it was the heart that was the starting point of fever, with body heat being central, viewed as an outcome of some processes (fermentation) in the blood.[4] During the sixteenth century, the whole discussion around the nature and characteristics of fever seemed to be more for the purpose of gaining knowledge than for

---

[4]During the sixteenth and seventeenth centuries, the terms 'fermentation', 'putrefaction', and 'effervescence' were used somewhat interchangeably by different scholars. During the early period, many scholars explained the processes in the blood during fever using the term 'putrefaction of humours', and this later became 'fermentation' or 'effervescence'. This is obvious from the sixteenth- and seventeenth-century descriptions of fevers dealt with by Lonie (1981) and Bates (1981).

practical purposes, and thus had little to do with the treatment per se. However, in the seventeenth century, the discussion of fevers shifted more towards prescribing the way that medicine should be practiced. This was also because many different views regarding treatment were struggling for legitimacy and orthodoxy (Bates 1981). It is in this context that the contribution of Thomas Willis becomes significant. Though his doctrine was not much different from earlier theories of fermentation in blood and the primacy of the heart, he also emphasised new ways of understanding the traditional treatment of fevers. His concern was not about the validity of treatment, but that whatever treatment was given should be given with a full understanding of its operations on the body (ibid.). This becomes evident from Willis' writing as cited by Bates: 'a medicine rashly administered is but casting a die for a man's life' (ibid: 59). This paved the way for the use of both traditional medicines and new ones like chemical remedies, provided that their use had been rationalised, which was a major issue among the Galenists and Paracelsians (Cartwright 1977: 17).

The shift of focus in the doctrine of fever towards everyday experiences of scholars mutually changed the collective knowledge as well as the condition itself. This is revealed by the fact that Northern Europeans and the British, who were the major contributors of fever literature, had experienced centuries of plague and at least two centuries of smallpox, typhus, typhoid, and dysentery by the seventeenth century (Bates 1981). Another important aspect of fevers dealt with by Willis as well as earlier by Fernel was 'rashes', again a clinical feature of the condition. Yet there was not much distinction in the way both dealt with rashes, as they were seen as signs of the 'degree of virulence' in most of the continued fevers (ibid: 66). In other words, rashes were seen as marks of severity. This is to say that though differences between rashes were never a serious concern, seventeenth-century authors increasingly wrote about smallpox and measles as if they were distinct diseases (ibid.). As for Bates (1981), this illustrates how the changing disease environment may have played a major role in the development of thought about fevers. Thus, a seventeenth-century understanding about fever was seen as a translation of a preeminently physiological disease to a clinical description. Going further, this was seen as a reflection of the acceptance of 'Baconian fashion', using Bates terminology (ibid. 69), whose culmination is seen in the work of Thomas Sydenham, who argued that the symptoms for similar diseases (species) remain the same among different persons (Reiser 1978: 9).

2.5 Practising Physicians' Knowledge of Fevers: An Eighteenth-Century Characteristic

During the last decades of the seventeenth century extending towards the early eighteenth century, the dominance of practising physicians and their theories over the pre-existing intellectual institutions of medical expertise were observed (Cunningham 1981; Geyer-Kordesch 1981). This could be possibly due to the upper hand of practising physicians in their ability to demonstrate efficacy through treatment. Thus, the prevalent principles[5] of treatment were questioned on the grounds of Sydenham's method of experimental basis, which envisages: 'the cure was found by confronting disease by skilled trial and error, rather than by working from within a theoretical understanding of physiology and pathology' (Cunningham 1981: 77). Three physicians were known for their contribution to fever theory during this period—Andrew Brown in Edinburgh following Sydenham's path, Cornelis Boentkoe in Holland, and Georg Ernst Stahl in Germany. Some commonalties can be identified in their approaches, as all of them were practising physicians and their theories on fevers were always tested within their daily practise of medicine. In other words, the physiology as well as the fever pathology per se became secondary, whereas disease descriptions based on prognosis and theory rooted in efficacy of the cure were the major focus. These physicians agreed on the opinion that nature has its own way of responding to any disease and that the task of the physician is either to assist or to facilitate this process depending on the stages of intervention (Cunningham 1981; Geyer-Kordesch 1981).

2.6 Classification of Fevers: The Primary Task During the Early Nineteenth Century

Later during the eighteenth century, Sauvages and Cullen following the work of Sydenham were engaged in the classification of diseases into classes, order, and genera (Reiser 1978: 9–10). Cullen, though recognised late, became well known during the early nineteenth century for his work on fevers. Cullen divided fevers into *periodic* and *continued,* and the latter was further sub-divided into *synocha, typhus,* and *synochus* (Smith 1981: 122). As Smith opines, Cullen's distinction is the same as that which classifies fevers as either *inflammatory, nervous,* or a third, mixed type neither purely inflammatory nor purely nervous (ibid.). Cullen's understanding of fevers and their connection to nerves was seen as an achievement of an open-minded physician who was keen in treatment. Following Sydenham, observing patterns in order to categorise fevers was a feature of seventeenth-century physicians as they were engaged in identifying epidemic patterns of similar kinds and associating them with the atmosphere (ibid.). Cullen learned from many of his forerunners and was more of a rationalist. Smith's (1981: 132) interpretation of Cullen's view of reasoning makes this evident:

> A physician used experience and reasoning in combination, the one supporting the other. Armed with analogies and the best understanding of physiological and pathological

---

[5]Fevers during Galenic times were found to occur due to four cause categories, viz. predisposing, external, antecedent, and immediate. Accordingly, treatment also comprised bleeding, vomiting, inciders (a medicine believed to have sharp particles that would cut up and allow the offending viscous fluid to be eliminated), and sweating. For more details, see Cunningham (1981).

processes the physician approached the bedside. He must always be aware of the limits of his theory *as the…* system is entirely defective [*emphasis added*].

Cullen furthered his study of fevers beyond classification and moved on to the stages of fever, viz. debility, chill, and heat, the first stage being in some sense the cause of the subsequent events (Bynum 1981). These stages defined fever both as a disease as well as a symptom when found in conjunction with other disorders. This was reflected in his practice of treating fever, where he elaborates:

> … Fever is a disease to be diagnosed by quizzing the patient about his feelings; by observing him for indications of shivering, sweating, and other manifestations of temperature change; and by carefully noting the sequence in which these events occur. (cf. ibid. 138)

At this juncture, it is interesting to note that despite the importance of body temperature in the description of fever, Cullen dismissed the role of the thermometer in measuring body heat, as the 'experience of the patient do not correlate very well with the numbers registered on the thermometer' (ibid. 138). Scholars consider the minimal use of thermometers by eighteenth-century doctors as more due to conceptual disagreement rather than technological ones (ibid., Reiser 1978: 110–120).

Moving on to the causes, Cullen identified *proximate* and *remote*, *external* and *internal*, and *predisposing* and *exciting*, encompassing prominent theories on causes and thereby linking them directly or indirectly to the physiological events of fever (Bynum 1981). This complex explanation of fever as compared to earlier ones was also reflected in his therapeutic practice. He considered a range of factors before deciding on any treatment, as reflected in his focus on climate, variety of fever, type of patients, and the stages of illness (ibid.). An understanding of fever as nature's effort to restore healthy equilibrium and the doctor's role being conceived of as only to assist nature were of less importance to Cullen. This is because he considered only the initial stage of fever as 'natural', and that it too needed to be countered medically as it would otherwise lead to *debility* or weakness (ibid. 139–140). To sum up, Cullen's classification of fevers was based more on the *clinical course* rather than on an aetiology that comprised a range of factors. He was also cautious of the difficulty in distinguishing between fevers, and therefore the diagnosis of fever was implicitly based on exclusion (ibid.), which is true even in current practice.

Cullen's remarkable contribution to identifying predisposing and exciting causes[6] as well as to the significant role that the doctor has to play in therapeutics influenced the need for isolation and special care for fever patients. The above understanding of fever transmission as well as significant cases reported from jails, ships, and cotton spinning factories, as well as in agricultural fields generated the

---

[6]Malnutrition and anxiety were considered predisposing causes whereas re-breathing expired air was seen as the major exciting cause. Also, the latter was strengthened by the frequent reporting of fevers from jails and ships, leading to the isolation of patients as a prerequisite for fever care. See also Pickstone (1992) and Bynum (1981).

idea of cleanliness, especially an obsession for fresh air as a means of prevention (Pickstone 1992; Bynum 1981). These factors together contributed to the setting up of 'fever wards' in the pre-existing general hospitals and later to fever hospitals during the late eighteenth century (Bynum 1981: 146).

2.7 Morgagni and 'Pathological Anatomy'

It was during the late eighteenth century that Morgagni observed pathological lesions in diseased bodies by opening up the corpses, which eventually became a method for disease identification (Reiser 1978:16; Foucault 1975). The general impact of this morbid anatomy on medicine was the shift from verbally oriented to observation-oriented[7] diagnosis (Reiser 1978). Foucault (1975: 181) interprets Morgagni's treatise on fevers as:

> ...an analysis of fevers based only on their symptoms, with no attempt at localisation, became not only possible but necessary: in order to provide the different forms of fever with a structure, organic volume had to be replaced by a space of division occupied only by signs and what they signify.

This expression by Morgagni shows how fever became understood as an exception to other diseases when it was found that bodily lesions, considered to be the feature of all diseases, were not necessarily always found in all kinds of fevers. This also resulted in an inquiry into the possibility of understanding fevers based on symptoms, which were usually seen as effects that could ultimately be traced back to bodily spaces (Foucault 1975: 182). This led to a shift in the classification of fevers from a system that was until then based merely on clinical symptoms to one based on symptoms and morbid anatomy, thereby institutionalising dissections in hospitals as a means for better understanding. On this Pickstone (1992: 141) elaborates:

> Surgeons were keen to dissect; in the services, as in civilian medical schools, mastery of the corpse was becoming a hallmark of the investigative doctor; the geography of the corpse was coming to rival the taxonomic spaces of nosologies, as the major means of 'placing' a disease.

Jewson (1976) called this a shift from 'bedside medicine' to 'hospital medicine', thereby changing the role of the early 'practitioner' to that of a 'clinician'.

Inspired by Morgagni's pathological anatomy that identified geographical divisions within the body and its organs, Bichat, a French physician, extended the analysis to the tissue level (Foucault 1975: 128–130). For Bichat, 'between the systems and tissues the organs appear as simple functional folds', entirely relative

---

[7]Up until the end of the eighteenth century, observation was mainly confined to the pulse as well as weakness of the patient and so on. Later, this shifted to observations (in a literal sense) that looked into the body (gaze). See also Jewson (1976) for clear distinction and Reiser (1978) for differences in patient examination during these two periods.

both in their roles and disorders (ibid.). In other words, the focus has changed from organ pathology to tissue pathology. This new approach not only resulted in a new categorisation of diseases based on lesions but also raised specific questions as to the very concept of disease in general and fevers in particular. First, does the lesion constitute the original three-dimensional form of disease or it is only the first visible manifestation of a hidden process? Second, is it necessary for all diseases to have lesions as a correlative within the body (ibid.)? The first question was not adequately addressed until Broussais' contribution, whose details will be dealt with later. Bichat addressed the second question (similar to the exception of fevers because of the absence of a lesion mentioned earlier) by treating certain kinds of fevers and nervous affections as non-lesional diseases, since there can be fevers *without* local lesions (essential) as well as *with* local lesions (sympathetic) (ibid.).

Returning to the first question, Broussais explains the mechanism of lesions in diseases through the case of fever and inflammation (lesion) as:

> ... a phenomenon involving two pathological layers at different levels and with different chronologies: first an attack on the functions, then an attack on the texture. Inflammation has a physiological reality that may anticipate anatomical disorganisation, which makes it perceptible to the eyes. (ibid: 186)

In other words, the functional disorders become primary and allow one to *perceive* the lesion, i.e. 'to make the observation of symptoms speak the very language of pathological anatomy' (ibid: 187). This is similar to theory-ladenness in observation where one can *see* only those things about which one is aware and the *ways of seeing* depend on the nature and kind of awareness (underlying theory). Thus, Broussais' contribution was in rediscovering the role of symptomatology that was side-lined during Bichat's work, since for the former it appears that symptomatology (knowledge about symptoms) is essential to the visibility of the lesions. Going further, Broussais argued that the absence of lesions is nothing but the ignorance of those who look for them, ignorance in terms of inadequate questioning (of symptoms) (ibid.). These efforts led to the disappearance of a *being* concept of disease, as the new explanation assumes the existence of disease *in space* before it is visible *for sight*, leading further to defining a *physiology of the morbid* phenomenon rather as normal and pathological anatomy (ibid. 188). This has also altered the causal aspect of diseases that has been a dominant area of inquiry since the seventeenth century, which was dismissed by Broussais in regarding 'the local space, the seat of the disease as also the causal space' (ibid.). To elaborate, the earlier notion of disease as a separate entity, with lesions as its genesis, was replaced by a new understanding, where the functional disorder (local space) of the system not only presupposed the presence of a disease, but also explained and predicted its nature and cause, which was validated by the lesion. Moreover, the medicine of diseases ultimately ceased to exist, thereby opening the path towards a medicine of pathological reactions, a structure of experience that dominated the nineteenth, and to a certain extent, the twentieth century (ibid.). In other words, it was this search for the physiology of the morbid phenomenon, later known as pathology, that generated a need to unravel the 'normal physiology' as an opposition to the former. This is what Canguilhem (1991: 42) argues, owing to Broussais and therefore to Comte, that '... pathological phenomena found in living organisms are nothing more than quantitative variations, greater or lesser according to corresponding physiological phenomena'.

2.8 Late Nineteenth- and Early Twentieth-Century Pathologisation on Fever

As mentioned before, Bichat's category of non-lesional diseases categorised fevers and nervous disorders together until the mid-nineteenth century (Foucault 1975: 175–176). Additionally, Broussais' approach was inadequate in addressing the ultimate origin (cause) of diseases, especially epidemics, thereby upholding the earlier doctrine that fevers were caused by a poison (Naraindas 1996: 8). This eventually led to a need to distinguish fevers and nervous disorders, resulting in the identification of the law of periodicity and a contagious characteristic as features specific to fevers (ibid.). The consequence of this was twofold. The first was the re-establishment of the pre-existent theory of contagion that attributed a kind of fever poison as the more general cause, which in turn could be an outcome of weather, overcrowding, or filth, which explained the *epidemic* character of the disease (ibid.). The second, concerning therapeutics, supported the earlier approach of allowing fevers to run their course, as symptoms were not treated as the cause of fever. This is owed to Broussais, who held that while in other diseases symptoms generally signified lesions, this was not always true for fevers (ibid.). The situation was more or less similar among physicians at the London fever hospital, who, though accepting of Broussais' doctrine on inflammation, also identified exhalations of the fevered bodies as the major means of propagation (Pickstone 1992). They saw these exhalations not as specific poisons, 'but as direct analogues of marsh miasma—as poisons arising from the decomposition of animal matter', which was the 'heart of the Chadwickian movement' in public health (ibid. 144).

This prevalent understanding of disease at the causal level provided space for the contagion or miasmatic theory of Chadwick (hygienists) that ultimately set the stage for Pasteur's germ theory, and for followers of Pasteur such as Robert Koch and Pettenkoffer (Cartwright 1977: 135–137). Here, it is highly possible that those diseases belonging to the categories of fever as well as other infectious diseases initially followed the miasmatic theory, and later, germ theory. This opens up infinite possibilities for discovering new causative organisms, be they microbes or viruses, and thus new diseases. Further extending the explanation of the ontology of diseases offered by Broussais, and expanded upon by Bernard, has resulted in a new field of specialisation, experimental pathology, based on the type of medical treatment performed (Canguilhem 1991: 58–64). Furthermore, Virchow's cell theory of 1858 not only replaced Bichat's theory on tissues as the building blocks of the body, but also ushered in a new technique for diagnosis: the laboratory (Cartwright 1977). It is highly possible that these perceptions of disease might have resulted in the treatment of non-infectious diseases, which are known to have multiple causal factors and hence are not necessarily looked for, as well as those infectious diseases whose causal factor could not be identified.[8] It could be that the extension of the above premise has created the biomedicine of the contemporary period, with an dependence on medical technology that is obvious from its power to define disease categories in technological terms. Having thus traced the history of fevers in the West, the history of fevers in the Indian subcontinent during the nineteenth and twentieth centuries will be examined below, in which it becomes clear that the former set the context for the latter.

2.9 History of Fevers in the Indian Subcontinent

Fevers have always been a common ailment in India. As mentioned before, several theories about fever existed in the West during the nineteenth century whose repercussions can be seen in the foundational understanding and conceptualisation of fever in the Indian sub-continent. Moreover, according to Rosenberg (1989: 14), in order to understand the framing of disease:

> ...[one] need to know more about the individual experience of disease in time and place, the influence of culture on definitions of disease and of disease in creation of culture, and the role of the state in defining and responding to disease ... understand the organization of medical profession and institutional medical care as in part a response to particular patterns of disease incidence.

Therefore, nineteenth-century India under British rule also acted as an experimental ground for the British in terms of the then prevalent theories of contagion and tropical diseases. Per the contagion theory, it was understood that living in tropical climates as well as in *unhygienic* living conditions together contributed to the process of putrefaction, thereby leading to morbidity (Naraindas 1996). Despite this notion, during the initial years of the nineteenth century the British believed that they could adapt to the Indian environment, especially the climate. Later during the epidemic of cholera this belief was shattered, with the British thereafter identifying the Indian conditions as *unhygienic* and *reservoirs of dirt and disease* (Harrison 1994: 48). Moreover, Indian medical systems like Ayurveda and Unani until the mid-nineteenth century shared with Western medicine a common notion of

---

[8]For infectious diseases the search for a causative agent resulted in the identification of a microbe in the case of cholera, dengue fever, leptospirosis, tuberculosis, avian flu virus, and so on. The list goes on unending, and the reality becomes clearer only through detailed study of the context of those discoveries of microbes similar to Latour's (1988) study on the *Pasteurization of France*. For non-infectious disease the search is not for microbes but for the abnormality in the physiology, a search that is armed by the available medical technology that redefines the abnormality and therefore defines diseases in technological terms, be them hypertension, diabetes, and so on. In other words, two kinds of disease definitions operate according to different logic despite the fact that the logic of disease management shows some similarities.

disease causation as a complex system of *exciting* and *predisposing causes* and rarely made reference to divine intervention, though moral conduct was considered an important factor (ibid.). It is in this context that the fevers in India during the nineteenth century will be examined.

Cholera was the major epidemic of the first half of the nineteenth century, whereas fevers and especially malaria were the major threat during the latter half. This was proven by reports from the Bombay presidency in 1856, which show that around 40 % of all deaths during the five-year period were due to fevers alone (Jaggi 2000: 151). It should be noted that until Laveran's discovery of the malaria parasite, malaria was thought even by the Europeans to be caused by 'miasma', arising from rotten vegetable matter (Harrison 1994; Jaggi 2000). The other fevers prevalent during this period were kala-azar, known by different names, viz. *kala-jwar, jwar-vikar, burdwan fever,* etc., and typhoid fever, also known as enteric fever. Earlier during the 1850s, several classifications of fevers were prevalent, of which *intermittent* and *remittent* were the broad clinical categories with similar causes but different degrees of the same kind of derangement (Jaggi 2000: 151). The essential difference between the two was that in the former there was complete cessation, whereas in the latter there was only an abatement of fever (ibid.). Belonging to the latter category, malaria's differential diagnosis was made based on seasonal consideration or on the possibility of the individual's previous exposure to malaria (ibid.).

TA third category included idiopathic fevers, also called ephemeral, common, continued, and so on, which were produced by changes in temperature, violent exercise, excitement of the mind, excess heat, and imperfect excretion (ibid.). Similar to the case of cholera (Singh 2001), there was staunch contradiction in the theories of causation and treatment in the case of malaria as well (Kumar 1998). Regarding fevers, it appears that not only was the theory on causation different but also the categories used were predominantly malaria-centric. The fact that during the mid-1800s both kala-azar and typhoid fevers were considered a type of malaria with exceptions, and also considering the *black water fever controversy*[9] during 1897 substantiates the above argument (Harrison 1994; Jaggi 2000). This becomes more obvious in an editorial on the aspect of fevers from the *Indian Medical Gazette*, published in 1872:

> There is no fact connected with the medical history of India more freely conceded by the most advanced thinkers in this country and indeed by any of those at home who take an interest in the matter that the obscurity which surrounds many forms of Indian fevers…Of all the causes, which have tended to obscure them, none appears to us to have been so powerful for evil as the too frequent use of the term malaria. In every attempt at scientific

---

[9]'Black water fever' or 'haemoglobinuria' was an illness during the mid-eighteenth century whose symptoms showed similarity to that of malaria and also turned the victim's urine dark red or black due to the toxins released into the blood stream. The London school headed by Manson considered this as a disease *sui generis*, whereas for another major group including Robert Koch, it was a form of quinine poisoning. This has prevented a significant population in India from taking quinine as a treatment for malaria. For more details, see Harrison (1994).

diagnosis we are met by the old bugbear malaria as either the cause of fever or it has imprinted its mark so indelibly that the original characters of the complaint are lost. (*Indian Medical Gazette*, 7, III, 1872, cf. Jaggi 2000: 152)

Despite this controversy, two methods of preventing the disease existed: the drainage or avoidance of swampy areas and the prescription of prophylactics provided by various cinchona preparations, most commonly quinine. Laveran's identification of the malaria parasite in the blood of malaria patients and Ross's later work that established the Anopheles mosquito as the vector of malaria, together with the *black water fever* controversy resulted in a malaria control programme predominantly comprised of mosquito eradication, anti-larval measures, and sanitation measures like the cleaning of drainage and avoidance of water collections owing to earlier sanitary traditions (Harrison 1994). Similar was the case with kala-azar, another disease that was confused earlier with malaria until its causative agent was found in 1904, and later, its transmission route. This time, however, the focus was predominantly on the treatment of affected cases rather than on the sanitation aspects. This change in focus could be due to the greater efficacy of treatment-based control measures as compared to the sanitary-based control measures carried out earlier, which were not successful as expected.

The case of typhoid fever, known then as enteric fever, was also identical to that of malaria in that there was strong objection to the discovery of a single micro-organism as the cause of the disease. Joseph Fayrer, the leading figure during this time criticised this attempt as follows:

The cause will probably not be revealed to anyone who searches with narrowed views. There is a great tendency in these days to trace all disease to a specific exterior cause, but we must not lose sight of the possibility of poisons auto-genetically developed…or of altered conditions of innervate. (Fayrer 1888, cf. Harrison 1994: 54.)

For Fayrer, germ theory was in itself inadequate to explain the cause of any disease, as more general environmental conditions were found that were more important than the germ. The sanitary commissioner from the government of India expressed his conviction that a specific germ theory was *inapplicable* to the history of enteric fever in India. This resulted in the propagation of sanitary measures as the major means for the control of enteric fever even after the discovery of the *typhosis* bacillus in 1884, thereafter known as typhoid fever, and even still after its confirmation (Harrison 1994: 56–58). This becomes obvious from the opinion of then sanitary commissioner with the Indian government, W.R. Rice: 'practically all bacteriologists agree[d] that bacillus [was] … a necessary factor in the causation of the disease, the question of how it was conveyed was still unresolved' (cf. Harrison 1994: 57).

The history of fevers in the Indian subcontinent during the nineteenth century raises certain issues. First, no uniform theory was yet agreed upon to explain the cause or the categories of fevers prevalent during this period, which was equally true in England. The dominance of malaria during this period might have led to many other fevers going unrecognised. Second, the germ theory of diseases faced staunch objections from the numerous sanitary commissioners as well as from the

Indian Medical Services, leading to a majority of the interventions during this period being ultimately targeted at sanitary activities. This could possibly have been due to the then-dominant paradigm of disease causation as well as the popular notion of *practical application* and *practical work* as being more important than the ambiguously understood microbial invasion leading to diseases. This dominance in the sanitary movement lasted until the early decades of the twentieth century. Another important feature of the twentieth century was that fevers were no longer 'seen' (to exist) as a disease but instead as a symptom for a range of diseases like malaria, typhoid, kala-azar, viral fever, and so on, the reason of which may have been the discovery of germs and thereafter the establishment of the germ theory. Thus, the twentieth-century history of fevers is in fact a history of discovery in terms of the causative organs of diseases with fever as a symptom, a field of inquiry that continues even today.

2.10 History of Public Health in Travancore[10]

Public health in Travancore can be traced back to the nineteenth century based on the diseases prevalent in what was then a princely state and by the interventions carried out by various institutions. Smallpox and cholera created a lot of havoc in Travancore, the intensity of which was at its peak during the late nineteenth century (Vinayachandran 2001: 49–54). However, smallpox vaccination has been in use in the state since 1813, thereby initiating the *preventive* approach within public health (ibid.). Initially, there was public dissent towards the use of vaccines due to the accumulation of puss at the vaccine site and the subsequent scar left there (ibid.). This problem was resolved, thereafter leading to the establishment of a vaccine department in 1865–1866, which underwent development several times with increasing numbers of staff and sub-departments (ibid.). It was reported that by the year 1935 around 71 % of the population was vaccinated in the region, which along with the reduction in the smallpox cases resulted in greater acceptance of public health activities (ibid., Panicker and Soman 1984: 50).

Epidemics of cholera were reported during the years 1819, 1822, 1837–38, and later in 1870, 1881, 1883, and 1892 (Kooiman 1991). Of these, the latter two epidemics took many lives, especially in northern Travancore (Vinayachandran 2001: 72–76). This ultimately led to the establishment of the sanitary department in 1895, despite the fact that fatality due to cholera was greater during the period after the establishment of the department (ibid.). The vaccine department that was under development also came under the administration of the sanitary department, with a sanitary commissioner in charge of both activities. The major functions of the

---

[10]Kerala before its formation consists of the princely states of Travancore, Cochin and Malabar. The state of Travancore covered the contemporary southern and central districts of Thiruvananthapuram, Kollam, Alappuzha, Pathanamthitta and parts of Kottayam.

department were vaccination and sanitation, the latter comprised of ensuring safe drinking water by digging new wells, cleaning old wells—involving use of chlorination when required—and introducing public health acts, especially to combat the plague and food adulteration (ibid. 43–45). The above set of activities also demonstrates the acceptance of public health as a separate field distinct from medicine, which reached its peak during the Second World War.

2.10.1   International Interventions in Public Health

The state of Travancore had plans to modernise its public health department since 1927 (ibid.) During the same period, the Rockefeller Foundation and the League of Nations were engaged in the field of public health activities worldwide and Travancore was identified as one of the possible destinations to receive their attention (ibid.). This, along with the state of Travancore's official request to modernise the existing public health activities, resulted in the submission of a report by Dr. W.P. Jackocks, the Foundation's representative who became adviser of the public health department from 1929 to 1933 (ibid., Kawashima 1998). Surveillance of hookworm infestation and its treatment and health education were the major recommendations of the Rockefeller Foundation, and subsequently resulted in the identification of 93 % of the population as infested with hookworm in the state; thereafter, the state implemented a Hookworm Eradication Programme (ibid., Panicker and Soman 1984: 34). It should be noted that the Rockefeller Sanitary Commission for the eradication of hookworm disease was founded in 1909 in the USA, whose concern was later extended to the rest of the world including Travancore (Kawashima 1998: 122–123). Additionally, there were recommendations from the health organisation of the League of Nations to select people from Travancore and send them for training at Johns Hopkins, Baltimore, and Harvard universities in order to make them capable of organising local health services (Vinayachandran 2001: 45). Thus, in September 1933, a new public health department was set up in which hookworm control was highlighted as the initial success story (ibid.). Some scholars critiqued the above interventions as 'the outcome of the concern towards the public health of the people in developing countries, a concern of the 'neo-colonialism' or the 'informal empire' which supplied raw materials to the developed world and also provided consumers for Western commodities' (Kawashima 1998: 123).

2.11   Medical Care in Travancore

By the end of the nineteenth century, Western medicine had gained acceptance among the public, thereby increasing the provisioning for various health institutions at different levels. Government-led initiatives established new hospitals for leprosy and mental illness, over which the state had authority, and also promoted private practice in rural areas (Vinayachandran 2001: 22–35). In addition to this, health institutions were set up by medical missions like the London Mission Society (LMS) (1838) as well as the Salvation Army (1885) (ibid. 85–95). In 1868, an Ayurvedic physician was appointed by the state in the civil hospital whose main duty was to identify the benefits of Ayurvedic medicine and to include it in the treatment regime (ibid. 72–76). However, the secondary status given to Ayurveda was changed by the end of nineteenth century, thereby initiating a movement for *revitalisation* that ultimately led to the setting up of the Ayurvedic departments in 1917–1918 (Panicker 1992; Kawashima 1998). Along with this, modern medicine was also supported by the government of Travancore, as reflected in a rise in the number of medical care institutions set up during the period. Only nine government medical institutions existed in the state of Travancore in 1863–1864, yet this grew to 27 hospitals and 26 dispensaries during 1915, and finally to 32 and 55, respectively, in 1939 together with 21 private health institutions financially supported by the government (Kawashima 1998: 117; Vinayachandran 2001: 30–35). Besides this, there were provisions for the free distribution of medicines as and when required through government machinery, of which the distribution in 1896 of quinine and chloroquine for malaria through post offices was the first such instance (ibid.).

After the success story of smallpox and hookworm treatments as well as the sanitary measures carried out, it was only in 1935–36 that cholera reappeared in the state, resulting in the deaths of around 6000 people (Vinayachandran 2001). Malaria was also reported in epidemic proportions during the same period in Travancore. For cholera, the interventions involved the chlorination of water sources together with vaccine distribution, whereas for malaria the surveillance centres took on the major task of distributing the treatment drug, quinine (ibid.). It is worth mentioning here that in 1931 a new division was started in the existing public health department to study malaria and filariasis, whose experts were from the school of tropical medicine in Kolkata (ibid. 78). Later in the next year, mosquito control measures were initiated in the state with the financial support of the Rockefeller Foundation, as the mosquito had been identified as the common vector for both malaria and filariasis (ibid.). After the epidemic of malaria in 1935–1936, a separate division for the control of malaria was set up that has since considerably checked the disease incidence (Panicker and Soman 1984).

2.11.1 Fevers in Travancore

Smallpox and cholera were the most prominent diseases to be reported in epidemic proportions in the state during the second half of the nineteenth century and proceeding into the early twentieth century. This could be due to the fact that plague, which was also an epidemic in other parts of India during this period, was not reported from the state. Additionally, the familiarity with smallpox and cholera made them easy to identify (Panicker and Soman 1984). It is an accepted fact that there was a steady decline of smallpox and cholera in the state, with a rapid pace for the latter especially after 1920–1921 (ibid.). Reports on the causes of death by the medical and public health departments of Travancore since the 1900s identified fevers as a major category along with cholera and smallpox. Of the total deaths, around 30 % were attributed to fever until the 1940s (Panicker and Soman 1984: 34). Since then, there has been a steady decline in deaths caused by fever, which is attributed by scholars to the decline in malaria cases (ibid.). Another disease that was prevalent in Travancore that involved fever symptoms was typhoid, then known as enteric fever. It was reported that the typhoid-paratyphoid A and B (T.A.B) vaccine was distributed through the public health laboratory, Thiruvananthapuram, during the 1940s, but the vaccine gained acceptance among the public only very slowly (Vinayachandran 2001).

2.11.2   Fever Care in Twentieth-Century Kerala

A brief outline on how fevers were dealt with in Kerala society during the mid-twentieth century can throw some light on the transformation of fever and fever care that has taken place in the recent period. During the nineteenth century, the benefits of Western medicine were felt in the state of Travancore, but these were essentially restricted to the family of the King while the common public was dependent more on the local practitioners who practiced local remedies (Vinayachandran 2001). It is obvious that the local practitioners themselves were not a homogeneous group, as they ranged from the present-day Ayurveds to naturopaths and other traditions. During the mid-nineteenth century, the order of treatment preference was first home remedies, then local remedies, and lastly, modern medicine (ibid.). Many of the treatments carried out by various systems of medicine were reportedly based on the symptoms and were effective, despite the fact that an understanding of the root cause was unknown (ibid.). During the early twentieth century, several systems of medicine prevailed, of which modern medicine was the last option.

Later, the establishment of the public health department that provided treatment for malaria, vaccine distribution for cholera, and other sanitary measures might have popularised modern medicine in the state. However, the worldwide acceptance of modern medicine as effective in tackling problems faced during the periods of World War I and II fuelled the domination of modern medicine in several places (Cartwright 1977). Despite this dominance of modern medicine by the mid-twentieth century, a range of home remedies was used to manage fevers. They included the intake of black coffee mixed with pepper and *chukku*, taking *kanji*' and *kurumulakurasam,*[11] and a variety of other preparations (Ramachandran 2000). Only if these failed did patients move on to seeking help from local practitioners, and finally to the allopathic system. In other words, it is obvious that fever was an illness that was managed effectively in homes in Kerala during the 1960s and 1970s. It should be noted that the fact that Kerala state was free of malaria until the mid-1960s also contributed to a situation in which fever was never a major threat (as it did not lead to death) for the population until the middle of the 1990s when it struck hard, as if it were an 'epidemic'.

2.12 History of Fevers and Public Health

The present chapter traces the history of fevers across the world from the sixteenth century to the current period. It is important to note that an understanding of fever as an illness—being as old as humankind—will then naturally involve the progression of humans and their interaction with diseases and medicine. During the sixteenth century an understanding of fever tended more towards description, whereas in the seventeenth century the search for causes began to result in the domination of the practising physician's interpretation based on experience, a feature that continued into the eighteenth century. It was during the late eighteenth and through the nineteenth century that the inquiry of fevers took a 'scientific' turn, in a time when anatomical interpretations dominated the field of medical understanding, and thus the understanding of fevers. The classification of fevers also expanded during this period. The modern understanding of fevers is an outcome of the engagement with the then dominant germ theory on one hand, and the uncertainty of those fevers whose causative agent could not be identified on the other. In the Indian context, the history of fevers is more a history of malaria, where other fevers were subsumed within the problem of malaria. This is true even today, as other diseases with fever as a symptom tend to get greater attention only in places where malaria is under control. The identification of different fevers in the states of Kerala and Tamil Nadu could therefore also be due to the negligible prevalence of malaria.

Another aspect that emerges from the Indian history of fevers is the public health profession's acceptance of the cardinal role of environment in preventing a range of diseases. The Indian public health sector, then dominated by the sanitary commissioners during the twentieth century, adopted sanitary measures as a way to prevent diseases despite the emergence and dominance of germ theory. This is an important orientation of public health, as even now there is a failure in the Indian context of public health to seriously engage with the environmental concerns of any

---

[11]*Chukku* is dried ginger, and *Kanji* is a mixture of rice and water prepared while making rice without draining the water. *Kurumulakurasam* is a preparation with tamarind, salt, tomato, pepper, and mustard, a favourite dish among those in southern India. When prepared to treat fever, the quantity of pepper will be increased slightly.

public health problem. This is evident in that the National Vector Borne Disease Control Programme (NVBDCP) considers the lack of cooperation by the environment department as a bottleneck to implementing vector control measures. The need to integrate environmental concerns into the Indian public health system is discussed elsewhere by the author (George 2016). The state of Kerala, too, saw numerous cases of malaria, cholera, and small pox until the early twentieth century, which then declined by the 1920s. Subsequently, the response to fevers was largely based upon home remedies and through the 'vaidyas' of Ayurveda at the local level, while modern medicine remained the last option. This treatment pattern is true even now for some groups in the states, a strategy that is also strongly proposed by some practitioners of alternative therapists as an option to be explored.

References

Atkinson, P. (1995). *Medical talk and medical work: The liturgy of the clinic.* London: Sage Publications.

Barnes, B. (1974). *Scientific knowledge and sociological theory.* London: Routledge and Kegan Paul.

Berg, M. (2004). Practices of reading and writing: The constitutive role of the patient record in medical work. In A. Ella, M. A. Elston, & L. Prior (Eds.), *Medical work, medical knowledge and health care.* UK: Blackwell.

Brown, P. J., Inhorn ,M. C., & Smith, D. J. (1996). Disease, ecology and human behaviour. In C. F. Sargent & T. M. Johnson (Eds.), *Medical anthropology: Contemporary theory and method* (revised edition, pp. 183–219). Connecticut, London: Praeger.

Bynum, W. F., & Nutton, V. (1981). Introduction. In W. F. Bynum & V. Nutton (Eds.), *Theories of fever from antiquity to enlightenment.*, Medical History Supplement No. 1, London: Wellcome Institute for the History of Medicine.

Canguilhem, G. (1991). *On the normal and the pathological.* New York: Zone Books.

Cartwright, F. F. (1977). *A social history of medicine.* London: Longman.

Casper, M., & Berg, M. (1995). Introduction: Constructivist perspectives on medical work: Medical practices and science and technology studies, *Science, Technology and Human Values*, special issue, *20*(4), 395–407.

Casper, M. J., & Morrison, D. R. (2010). Medical sociology and technology: Critical engagements. *Journal of Health and Social Behaviour, 51*(S), S120–S132.

Clarke, A. E., Shim, J. K., Mamo, L., Ruth, F., & Fishman, J. R. (2003). Biomedicalization: Technoscientific transformations of health, illness, and US biomedicine. In G. Albrecht, R. Fitzpatrick, & S. Schrimshaw (Eds.), *Handbook of social studies in health and medicine* (pp. 442–445). London: Sage.

Cornad, P. (2007). *The medicalization of society: On the transformation of human condition into treatable disorders.* Baltimore: Johns Hopkins University Press.

Engel, G. L. (1977). The need for a new medical model: A challenge for biomedicine. *Science, 196* (4286), 129–136.

Engelhardt, T., Jr. (1976). Ideology and etiology. *The Journal of Medicine and Philosophy, 1*(3), 256–268.

Foucault, M. (1975). *The birth of the clinic: Archaeology of medical perception.* New York and London: Vintage Books.

Fox, R. C. (1989). *The sociology of medicine, a participant observer's view.* Engelwood Cliffs, NJ: Prentice Hall.

Fox, R. C. (2000). Medical uncertainty revisited. In G. L. Albrecht, R. Fitzpatrick, & S. C. Scrimshaw (Eds.), *Handbook of social studies in health and medicine*. London: Sage.

George (2016) Health care norms under universal health care (UHC) for Maharashtra: Relieving illness and ensuring public health, *Journal of Health Management*, 18, 4.

Good, B. J. (1994). *Medicine, rationality and experience, an anthropological experience*. Cambridge: Cambridge University Press.

Hampton, J. R., Harrison, M. J. G., Mitchell, J. R. A., Prichard, J. S., & Seymour, C. (1975). Relative contributions of history-taking, physical examination and laboratory investigation to diagnosis and management of medical outpatients. *British Medical Journal, 2*, 486–489.

Jewson, N. D. (1976). The disappearance of the sick man from medical cosmology 1770–1870. *Sociology, 10*, 225–244.

Jutel, A. (2009). Sociology of diagnosis: A preliminary review. *Sociology of Health & Illness, 31*(2), 278–299.

Lupton, D. (1994). *Medicine as culture: Illness, disease and the body in the western societies*. London: Sage.

McCullough, L. (1981). Thought-styles, diagnosis, and concepts of disease: Commentary on Ludwick Fleck. *The Journal of Medicine and Philosophy, 6*, 257–261.

Petersdorf, R. G. (1974). Disturbances of heat regulation. In M. M. Wintrobe, G. W. Thorn, R. D Adams, E. Braunwald, K. J Isselbacher, & R. G. Petersdorf (Eds.), Harrison's principles of internal medicine (7th ed., pp. 48–62). New Delhi: Tata McGraw Hill.

Reiser, J. S. (1978). *Medicine and the Reign of technology*. Cambridge, UK: Cambridge University Press.

Rosenberg, C. (2002). The tyranny of diagnosis, specific entities and individual experience. *The Millbank Quarterly, 80*(2), 237–260.

Samson, C. (1999). The physician and the patient. In C. Samson (Ed.), *Health studies, a critical and cross cultural reader*. UK: Blackwell Publishers.

Temkin, O. (1964). Historical aspects of drug therapy. In P. Talaly (Ed.), *Drugs in our society*. Baltimore: Johns Hopkins University.

Vishwanathan, S. (1997). *A carnival for science, essays on science, technology and development*. Calcutta, New Delhi: Oxford University Press.

White, K. (2002). *An introduction to the sociology of health and illness*. London: Sage.

Chapter 3
Institutionalising Fever Epidemics and Fever Care in Contemporary Kerala

Abstract During the mid-1990s, the south Indian state of Kerala witnessed a wave of 'fever epidemics', to for which *fever clinics* were established in an attempt to combat them. This chapter demonstrates how *fever* was framed as an epidemic and became institutionalised as a *disease,* and then examines the context of establishing *fever clinics* as a *cure.* A detailed ethnography of these fever clinics demonstrates how the institutionalisation of disease and cure happens *through practice* within the microcosm of a clinic. It is argued that the institutionalisation of fever as a disease happened through two acts: first, through the discourse on fevers produced at the societal level by interactions among the health professionals, the media, organisations representing various systems of medicine, and the people; second, in the course of rendering fever care at the fever clinic, which involved diagnosis and treatment. This chapter maintains that the institutionalisation of disease and cure happens in accordance with the dominant system of medicine. However, the processes at the fever clinic demonstrate that fever care is not necessarily based on a theoretical understanding of physiology and pathology as claimed by the allopathic medical fraternity—rather, it is a process of confronting disease by skilled trial and error. The chapter concludes by cautioning against the power of institutionalisation that not only generates a threat about fevers but also limits alternatives for tackling them.

Keywords Discourse analysis · Fever epidemics · Fever clinics · Institutionalizing fever · Plural systems · Multi-site ethnography

3.1 Fevers as Discourse

Fever is conceptualised as an illness that acquires meaning depending on the actors and the context involved, and whose meaning will be interpreted based on the discourse in which it is embedded. This chapter examines fevers as understood by

---

Portions of this chapter are also to be found in Contribution to Indian Sociology 2011, 45(3), 373–397.

the medical fraternity, laymen, public health experts, the media, and so on, in order to situate their understanding in their respective contexts. The everyday activities of individuals produce certain notions about fever that, in turn, can also determine everyday actions regarding the distress associated with fever along with relevant government policies. Thus, fever is understood as a discourse within Kerala society where the very notion of fever among various social groups has to be historically and culturally situated within the prevalent societal discourse on health, illness, and medicine. For instance, fever for the medical fraternity could be largely influenced by the prevalent discourse on medicine, in which fever may be treated as a symptom marked by a physiological indication of elevated body temperature (greater than 98.4 °F). In comparison, the notion of fever for a person affected with the illness can be that which interferes with his/her day-to-day behaviour and action as part of daily life. It is interesting to note that the media as well as health professionals consider fever as an epidemic that can cause death during outbreaks.

3.2   Discourse Analysis as Theory and Method

Discourse analysis provides a tool for analysing this kind of complexity, especially in understanding health and illness within the prevalent medical discourse (Yardley 1997). *Discourse* is defined as a particular way of talking about and understanding the world (or an aspect of the world). This approach considers human ways of talking as not merely a neutral reflection of their world, identities, and social relations, but as playing an active role in creating and changing them (Jorgensen and Phillips 2002). As such, the act of talking is not a passive act of articulation but an active one that can change the world by interpreting the world and its events differently. Discourse analysis is carried out with the following assumptions. *First*, *reality* can be accessed only through categories, resulting in understanding reality as that which is produced during the process of categorising the world. This is not to say that reality is *out there* and needs to be discovered; rather it is the product of the prevalent discourse and is produced in the process of interpretation. *Second*, these views and knowledge about the world and their categories are historically and culturally specific and situated. This implies the existence of a historical and cultural identity attached to the events and the analyses, as the identities are contingent and always subject to change. *Third*, an understanding of the world is accomplished through social processes and can lead to contention due to various ideas and knowledge about the same event. This implies that there can be multiple interpretations of the same event, along with common truths as well as dissension between truth and false claims that occur through social processes. *Finally*, human action must be seen as that determined by a social understanding of the world, and hence having social consequences. In other words, social action is influenced by social perceptions, and changing social perceptions can thus change social actions (ibid. 5–6). Therefore, discourse analysis is not merely a method of data analysis—rather, it is a theoretical and methodological whole in which there are theoretical assumptions as well as specific methodological guidelines and techniques for approaching a problem. In other words, using Jorgensen and Phillips' (2002: 7) terminology there is an *intertwining of theory and method in discourse analysis*, where the basic premises will always remain as a pretext for any method of empirical study.

Thus, diverse notions of fever have to be seen as that having both a historical and cultural genealogy, where the understanding of disease at different points of time together with the evolution of medicine and, more importantly, human experience with distress, would also have influenced the contemporary notions about fever. In order to understand the various notions of fever, there is an inevitable need to examine the social, economic, political, and cultural context prevalent in the society, where the shaping of people's perceptions is very much a product of the prevalent structures. Yardley (1997: 7) therefore opines that any attempt to understand people's notions about health and illness should:

> ...consider their socio-cultural functions and connotations, and the ways in which these may be influenced by class, age, gender or ethnic background, by macro-level social policies or micro-level patterns of social interaction and by representations of health in the media in medical discourse, or in casual conversation.

Thus, discourse analysis offers an adequate scope for a contextual understanding of fever that provides ample space for explaining various events, historical, political, social, and cultural aspects related to the illness that facilitate better understanding.

The present chapter examines how multiple discussions about fevers take place at different sites, and different institutions interpret the illness from their own perspectives. The anxiety about the threat of fevers has resulted in diverse responses across groups of people. One such response of the state government to this anxiety has taken the form of establishing fever clinics. This has transformed the status of fever from that of a symptom to that of a disease, which is in contrast to the dominant biomedical discourse that regards fever only as a symptom characterised by an elevation of body temperature, a physiological defensive response to an underlying disease, or any external pathogenic attack (Kohl et al. 2004; Mackowiak 1998; Mackowiak et al. 1997). How this shift has occurred is examined by tracing the way in which fever became institutionalised as an epidemic in Kerala. The chapter is divided into four sections. The first contextualises the discourse on fevers in Kerala by briefly describing those epidemic diseases which feature fever as a major symptom. The second section focuses on 'fever talk', the way fever is discussed among doctors, other health professionals, the media, and the public. It shows how these interactions engender fear of fever, thereby discursively framing it as an epidemic to be managed by the establishment of fever clinics in the state. The third section examines how the process of diagnosis and treatment in the fever clinics reinforces the institutionalisation of fever as an epidemic. The concluding section discusses the implications of this process of institutionalisation for a more effective understanding of disease and wellbeing.

I

3.3   Disease Profile of Contemporary Kerala

Illnesses like 'viral fevers, upper and lower respiratory tract infections, simple cough and runny nose' are generally classified as fevers (Kunjhikannan and Aravindan 2000: 15; Panicker and Soman 1984), as are the symptoms of diseases like malaria, typhoid, and measles. Fevers as a group have always constituted a major category in the morbidity profile of Kerala, accounting for more than 50 % of the total illnesses reported during the 1980s and mid-1990s (Kannan et al. 1991; Krishnaswami 2004; Kunjhikannan and Aravindan 2000). By 1953, the incidence of malaria in Kerala was under control and hence, the contribution of fevers as a proportion of other causes of death was reduced (Panicker and Soman 1984). However, after 1969, the number of malaria cases gradually increased again (Remadevi and Dass 1999). Since the mid-1990s, in addition to malaria, Kerala has experienced outbreaks of Japanese encephalitis, leptospirosis, dengue, chikungunya, and what is generically described as 'viral fever'. Their scale, contagious nature, and sometimes fatal consequences led to these diseases being categorised as 'epidemic fevers'.

3.3.1   Epidemic Fevers

Japanese encephalitis was reported in epidemic proportions in Kerala during 1996, 1997, and 1998 with 32, 7, and 14 deaths, respectively, after which there was no significant number of cases (see Table 3.1). It was the incidence of other fevers including leptospirosis, dengue fever, and viral fever that seems to have triggered the establishment of fever clinics in the state. Though the causative agent of leptospirosis[1] was identified for the first time using laboratory tests in 1987, doctors claim to have treated cases of leptospirosis since 1982.[2] No uniform diagnostic procedure has yet been established for the disease. Diagnosis of leptospirosis is a major problem as it has symptoms similar to dengue, Japanese encephalitis, malaria, and typhoid. Thus, it tends to be under-reported since many institutions do not track its prevalence,[3] leading to a gap in the consolidated data (George 2007b).

Dengue fever was first reported in 1997, and since 2001, Kerala has been reporting cases every year, with the largest number (3861) reported in 2003. The

---

[1]Leptospirosis is also known as Weil's disease, mud fever, trench fever, rice-field fever, cane cutter's fever, and swineherd's disease. These names indicate that the disease was initially associated with occupational groups. The disease is transmitted among humans by domestic and wild animals; rats are the major carriers.

[2]Personal communication, Head of the Infectious Disease Unit, Kottayam Medical College, Kottayam, Kerala.

[3]As part of the surveillance effort of the government, certain diseases when treated at any hospital have to be reported to the district medical authorities. Those considered mandatory for reporting are called 'notifiable' diseases and their list is periodically reviewed by the government.

Table 3.1 Number of cases and deaths reported due to various diseases during 1996–2010

Disease	Year	1996	1997	1998	1999	2000	2001	2002	2003	2004	2005	2006	2007	2008	2009	2010
Malaria	Cases	Was not tracked and reported until 2006										2130	1927	1804	2046	2299
	Deaths											6	6	3	6	7
JE	Cases	106	61	199	0	0	0	0	0	0	0	14	2	9	23	20
	Deaths	32	7	14	0	0	0	0	0	0	0	1	1	0	9	5
Leptospirosis	Cases	–	–	342	763	1174	2582	2928	2162	2356	1366	1821	1359	1305	1237	1016
	Deaths	–	–	64	65	87	129	199	97	220	101	104	229	136	107	85
Dengue	Cases	–	14	0	0	0	74	163	3861	1622	1028	1019	657	733	1425	2597
	Deaths	–	4	0	0	0	0	1	35	19	8	5	11	3	6	17
Viral Fever	Cases	–	–	–	–	–	–	–	1549	1292	2145	1,655,329	Data was not consolidated after this			
	Deaths	–	–	–	–	–	–	–	–	51	132	74				
Chikungunya	Sus	Only began data consolidation in 2006										70,731	24,052	24,685	13,349	1708
	Con.											54	1092	470	597	210

Source Directorate of Health Services, Thiruvananthapuram, IDSP Kerala

lack of a standard disease definition has been a major issue for dengue as well. Private and public hospitals follow different methods of diagnosing dengue fever. These conflicting practices became apparent when the number of cases and deaths reported in 2003 was halved (1622) in the following year. As a district medical officer pointed out, 'Cases reported from private hospitals were also included in 2003; this stopped in 2004 as several false positive cases were reported from private hospitals which used only the platelet count as a basis for the diagnosis of dengue fever'.[4] The likelihood that the incidence of dengue fever was over-reported was supported by the fact that only a small percentage of blood samples tested for the dengue virus among suspected cases showed the presence of virus.[5] It could be argued that private hospitals tend to report a range of fevers as dengue fever even when that may not be the case, as it is a more 'marketable' event, and the fear around its severity can be exploited to justify more costly medical interventions.

It is more likely, however, that what is often diagnosed as dengue could be a range of unidentified viral fevers. This has been a feature of fevers, as is obvious from the statement, 'Most undiagnosed acute febrile infectious diseases are probably viral and remain undiagnosed because diagnostic methods are unavailable or cumbersome' (Petersdorf 1974: 57). For practical clinical purposes, an 'exclusion principle' is widely used to diagnose viral fever. As the head physician of the infectious diseases unit in one of the medical colleges in Kerala explained:

> ...a patient with fever will be asked questions and, based on the specific symptoms, lab tests will be prescribed pertaining to the diagnosis of typhoid, malaria, measles, chicken pox and leptospirosis. Once these diseases are ruled out through laboratory investigations, it is assumed that the patient is suffering from infection and, as it is believed that the majority of infections are caused by virus, the fever is classified as viral fever.

The physician also described the standard procedure in such cases:

> For viral fevers, the principle of treatment is 'symptomatic treatment' where, rather than eliminating the cause of the illness [as in the case of bacterial diseases], medicine that can reduce symptoms will be prescribed and in due course the body will resist the disease.

The 'exclusion principle' means that, in situations where malaria is no longer endemic and where the absence of rashes implies the elimination of measles and chicken pox as a likely possibility, physicians are likely to arrive at a diagnosis of viral fever. This can occur even when the illness could be a respiratory infection or a simple cold. Viral fever was categorised as a *notifiable* disease by the state only in

---

[4]In most private hospitals, dengue fever is diagnosed solely on the basis of the patient's blood platelet count. Physicians say that while a low platelet count does occur in the case of dengue fever, it can also be caused by anaemia or the use of certain drugs, especially steroids. For more details, see 'Myths Prevail in Society about Dengue', *The Hindu*, October 1, 2006.

[5]In the year 1997, of the 116 cases examined from Kottayam district, only 14 cases were confirmed in laboratory tests. During 2001, 70 probable cases were confirmed out of 877 reported from the four districts. For more details, see Kalra and Prasittisuk (2004).

2004, and by 2006 there was a tremendous increase in the number of cases reported (See Table 3.1). It would appear that physicians in government hospitals and clinics did not try to distinguish dengue cases from other viral fever, arguing that 'the intervention remains the same whether it is viral fever or dengue fever and it is the concern of the epidemiologist to distinguish between the two and not the clinician's'. Incidentally, it is also said that the treatment protocol for early stages of dengue and chikungunya are also similar (Ramachandran 2006). Even the categorisation of chikungunya as suspected and confirmed by the government is an indication of the medical uncertainty that exists in its diagnosis.

3.3.2 Reporting Fevers

The resemblance between different fevers and their common treatment protocols and the diverse diagnostic procedures followed across hospitals creates a puzzling situation leading to an absence of uniform disease definition, a prerequisite for any epidemiological analysis. Hence, there is a greater possibility for conflicting diagnoses, resulting in under-reporting of some fevers and over-reporting of others. This could also be due to the organisational constraints within the public health reporting system (Banerji 1984). The gap between diagnosis, treatment, and cure is evidenced by the large proportion of patients who were cured of their illness despite the physician's failure to arrive at a confirmed diagnosis.[6] Of the 151 fever patients followed in this study, only 14 % had a final confirmed diagnosis and 22 % had a suspected diagnosis; the majority (64 %) were categorised only at the symptom level without any diagnosis at all (George 2007a). However, several practising physicians do not see this as a shortcoming, pointing out that diagnosis at the symptomatic level is usually sufficient for medical treatment, especially for diseases like leptospirosis. These factors contribute to the creation of a generic disease category, namely 'fever', the discourse around which is examined in the next section.

II

---

[6]For a confirmed diagnosis, it is necessary that the illness identified by a physician after examining a case should fit into the pre-existing symptom and disease categories of the system of medicine practised by the physician. The 'Protocol for Syndrome of Fever', a draft document prepared by the Directorate of Medical Education, Government of Kerala, to guide 'fever management' through surveillance and treatment protocols, advises that diagnoses be classified as Suspected, Probable, and Confirmed.

3.4   Fever Talk: The Discursive Production of a Disease

The rise of fever cases in the state led the Department of Health Services to organise meetings with ministers, public health professionals, and other government officials. The proposed public health interventions included effective waste disposal, vector control measures, and more importantly, establishing fever clinics across the state.[7] It was found that until 2002 the major cause among fevers was leptospirosis, except for during the outbreak of encephalitis during 1996–1998. However, a few cases of dengue were also reported in the state during 2002. Thus, dengue and Japanese encephalitis joined the ranks of leptospirosis as notifiable diseases. In another meeting chaired by the Chief Minister in February 2003 on 'Intersectoral Approach and Prevention and Control of Leptospirosis and other Communicable Diseases', it was decided that each District Medical Officer (DMO) be allotted an amount of Rs. million for the prevention and management of communicable diseases, with Rs. 200,000 each to the government medical colleges. The proposed interventions focused on establishing procedures for diagnosing and reporting cases from different public and private hospitals in the state, as well as vector control measures based on sanitation and larvicidal measures along with Information, Education, and Communication (IEC).[8] In a meeting held on July 29, 2003, it was reported that viral fever was present in epidemic proportions in the northern districts of Kannur and Kasargod. A series of eight meetings of the newly formed state-level Crisis Management Committee (CMC) held on July 11–29, 2003, against the backdrop of rising numbers of dengue cases in the state, called for the formation of district-level CMCs with the District Collector at their helm and functioning extended to the ward level. The CMC recommended prompt reporting of diseases (especially from private hospitals) following a specified format, and assigned to the DMO of each district the responsibility of consolidating data from private hospitals and sending it to the Directorate of Health Services (DHS). A related decision was to distribute diagnostic kits received from the World Health Organisation (WHO) to all public health labs at the district level.[9]

A preliminary epidemiological investigation report on the outbreak of leptospirosis and dengue fever that had occurred during July 2003 was submitted in October 2003. The report recommended that regular fever clinics be set up in medical colleges, district hospitals, CHCs, and primary health centres (PHCs). This recommendation came after the successful strategy of organising camps and fever

---

[7]This study is confined to a review of meetings held during 2002–2004, until the state government officially declared the establishment of fever clinics on May 24, 2004 (Minutes of the meetings on communicable diseases held on May 24, 2004, with the Minister for Health as convenor, also see *The Hindu* dated May 25, 2004).

[8]Minutes of the meeting on Intersectoral Approach and Prevention and Control of Leptospirosis and other Communicable Diseases, held on February 3, 2003, with the Chief Minister as the president.

[9]Minutes of the State Level Crisis Management Committee on Communicable Disease meetings, July 11–29, 2003.

clinics, usually in conjunction with existing health centres and occasionally separate, depending on the quantum of cases reported. The first fever clinic was started on June 25, 2003, at Vithura in Thiruvananthapuram district after a five-year-old boy died in the area. Later, when fever cases were reported in large numbers, several fever clinics (known as 'monitoring cells' in some places) were started in public health institutions ranging from CHCs to district hospitals. The major tasks were to identify fever cases, manage them effectively, and report them promptly to the district authorities.

Public health experts evaluated the situation in the state in a Meeting on Communicable Diseases, the first of its kind, held on February 3, 2004, with the Principal Secretary of Health as Chairman. Based on an earlier report about procedures to be followed for investigating an epidemic, a Protocol for the Syndrome of Fever was prepared on how to manage fever cases with the major focus on disease reporting, diagnosis, and management (see Footnote 6). This 10-page report, drafted during the epidemic of 2003, remains a key document on fever case definition and its prevention. The description of fever as a 'syndrome' in the document indicates its transition from being a symptom of various diseases to a bodily condition characterised by certain signs and symptoms similar to other disorders like AIDS, Down syndrome, and Guillain-Barré syndrome. In other words, fever is assigned a position somewhere between a symptom and a disease, if symptom and disease can be seen as the two ends of a continuing spectrum. The report provides details on how surveillance needs to be carried out by classifying cases as *suspected, probable,* and *confirmed,* depending on clinical signs, supporting evidence from blood tests and chances of contact with a confirmed case. The document provides guidelines on the reporting procedures to be followed and lists measures for preventing and controlling an outbreak. The major focus of these measures is on vector control: mosquitoes in the case of dengue, Japanese encephalitis, and malaria, and rodents in the case of leptospirosis. The second part of the document deals with the clinical and laboratory criteria for the diagnosis and management of dengue fever, Japanese encephalitis, and leptospirosis with a reminder to physicians as to the protocol to be followed in case of an epidemic.

3.4.1   Response from the Media and the Public

While the government records suggest a calm and methodical response to the epidemic, the tone of the media reports was not the same. The media spotlighted fever cases and criticised the government, pointing out problems such as the paucity of doctors, the lack of adequate treatment at the hospitals, and poor hospital waste management as directly or indirectly responsible for the epidemic.[10] Since the

---

[10]Similar factors were identified during the plague epidemic in Surat and the dengue epidemic in Delhi (Addlakha 2001; Shah 1997).

1990s, local newspapers published a column on *'panimaranangal'* (deaths due to fever) during and immediately after the monsoons. Television channels as well as vernacular magazines highlighted the risks of fever and the precautions to be taken. This coverage deepened the public's sense of fevers as an epidemic to be feared.

Some reports on deaths due to fever that appeared in the newspapers during the epidemic reveal the uncertainty and confusion prevalent among physicians and the public:

> Arjun, a fourth standard student of the Sarvodaya Vidyalaya, Nalanchira, was admitted to the SAT Hospital on Monday following symptoms of dengue fever. He died of 'bleeding and shock' this morning [Wednesday] while under treatment in the ICU. The hospital Superintendent, K. Rajamohan said Arjun, son of a staff nurse of the hospital and a resident of Burma Road, Kumarapuram, had 'clinical dengue as there was bleeding'. The boy, who had been attending school, developed fever on Friday evening and was taken to the hospital. Following this, he was under treatment at home. He was rushed to the hospital yesterday after he showed symptoms of dengue fever.[11]

In another report:

> An MCH official said that two youth from Nedumangad had been hospitalised in a critical state with high fever. One, who was 22 years old, died within hardly 10 min of being admitted to the hospital, while the other, who was 18 years old, succumbed after battling for life for three hours in the ICU. The third patient, a 19-year-old girl from Sreevarahom area in the city, died while under emergency care in the Medical Intensive Care Unit (MICU). She had arrived with tell-tale signs of an end-stage dengue attack. Clinicians, however, were reluctant to classify the infective cause of the deaths, as serological confirmation could not be obtained in any of the cases. Doctors said the two youth from Nedumangad appeared to have suffered from severe broncho-pneumonia and had difficulty in breathing.[12]

> Even a death reported today in Kollam has been formally described by the health authorities as 'suspected rat fever'. The fact that the medical authorities cannot identify what precisely caused a person's death, especially in a tense situation in which an epidemic is raging, only exposes the total inefficiency on the part of the health authorities in dealing with the situation.[13]

As discussed above, valid diagnosis is difficult when the symptom of fever can be caused by one of a range of diseases. Once an afflicted person dies, the task of determining which disease was responsible is even harder. Without explaining the medical complexity of the issue, media reportage repeated medical terms such as 'suspected' and 'clinical signs' to convey the expert and authoritative character of these diagnoses and, in the process, suggests a medically-sanctioned scenario of dramatic death and disease (see Fox 1957, 2000). In the absence of adequate evidence, media columns like 'panimaranangal' aggravated public perceptions of

---

[11]*The Hindu*, June 28, 2003.

[12]*The Hindu*, June 20, 2003.

[13]*Indian Express*, June 28, 2003.

the threat from fevers.[14] In order to understand the realistic scenario of the reports on *panimaranangal,* one such case was traced back to its details: the story of a 15-year-old girl reported in the newspaper to have died of fever. On detailed inquiry it was found that fever was one of the symptoms present during the girl's death, but she also had a history of heart defects and the cause of death was inconclusive according to the doctor who treated her. Fears about viral fever were also amplified in the clinics established to treat them when physicians coined the category of *vishapani* (poisonous fevers) to distinguish viral fever from other kinds. This physician-created category, devised ostensibly for patients who may not under- stand, was internalised and became a part of the public discourse such that patients began referring to their illnesses as *vishapani.* Thus, the doctor–patient interaction became a site of knowledge production that aggravated, rather than calmed, patients' anxiety about their illnesses.

3.4.2   Fever Talk in Plural Systems of Medicine

If the discourse on fevers pitted government doctors and public health authorities against a fearful public and sensationalising media, it also sparked off contestation between institutions representing different systems of medicine, viz. the Indian Medical Association (IMA), which represents practitioners of the allopathic (Western biomedicine) system, and the Organisation of Government Homoeopathic Medical Officers of Kerala (OGHMOK), which represents the homoeopathic sys- tem. In the wake of an epidemic, the IMA conducted a survey among 1040 high school students and a street sample of 528 people from Thiruvananthapuram city to study the extent of the epidemic and the efficacy of homoeopathic medicines. The study noted the higher-than-usual prevalence of fever and diagnosed it as dengue fever caused by ineffective vector control measures. The study also criticised people's misplaced reliance on homoeopathic drugs as a preventive measure, claiming that those who took these medicines were also reported to develop fever as well as side effects.[15]

In response to this, the OGHMOK challenged the IMA's diagnosis of dengue and urged the state government to conduct a probe into the 170 deaths that were attributed to dengue fever. Dr V.A. Nassirudheen, president of the OGHMOK, rebutted the charge that homoeopathic medicines were not effective against viral and dengue fever. He asserted that only homoeopathy could offer medicines to prevent the fever, which had been raging in the state for two months.[16] This conflict

---

[14]Also see newspaper reports on epidemics during 2002–2004, cited in www.kerala_ epidemicsblogspots.com/2003-09-1_keralaepidemics_archive.html. Accessed March 27, 2005.

[15]*The Indian Express,* July 14, 2003.

[16]*The Indian Express,* July 25, 2003.

was also reflected in a subsequent meeting of the state-level CMC.[17] The committee recommended that a scientific study on the effect of homoeopathic and ayurvedic preventive medicines be conducted. However, financial constraints and dwindling interest meant that this was not done.[18]

In this controversy, the state and the media unquestioningly sided with the dominant allopathic system, despite the failure of this system to come up with an effective way of diagnosing or treating different kinds of fevers. In doing so, they also dismissed the possibility of arriving at any alternative or more effective therapies based on other medical systems.[19] The perceived failure of homoeopathic medicine in the case of what biomedical practitioners diagnosed as dengue fever indicates that the epistemological differences between the two systems are assimilated into an institutionalised asymmetry. Questions of evidence and efficiency, according to Naraindas:

> … are central to the interplay between biomedical and other medical traditions, since objective tests and measures in biomedicine are accepted as the only legitimate 'evidence' of cure, but these do not necessarily accord either with the premises of these other traditions or with patients' subjective perceptions of well-being. (Naraindas 2006: 2658)

The uncritical acceptance of biomedicine by the government and the media not only determines the availability of medical services but also influences people's decisions about using alternative therapies. With the institutional weight of the state and the authority of the media supporting biomedicine and its claimed monopoly of knowledge of health and illness, even those people who are getting relief through alternative systems can become more doubtful and anxious. Yet, biomedicine remains the dominant system despite its inability to adequately diagnose and treat fevers.

3.4.3 Establishment of Fever Clinics

The circulating discourse of 'fever talk' provided the context within which a new health minister who took charge in February 2004 felt compelled to act decisively.[20] Immediately upon his assuming the role, cases of malaria were reported from the Valiathura fishing community at Thiruvananthapuram, a highly endemic area for malaria in the state from which cases had been regularly reported since

---

[17]Minutes of the state level Crisis Management Committee on Communicable Disease meeting held on August 13, 2003, 6th recommendation.

[18]Minutes of the state-level Crisis Management Committee on Communicable Disease meeting held on August 20, 2003.

[19]For historical accounts of institutional support for Western biomedicine, see Frankenberg (1981); Panikkar (1992).

[20]The previous minister was removed from his post on charges that he planned to lease out government medical college campuses to private companies. *The Hindu,* June 29, 2003.

1997 (Remadevi and Dass 1999). By February 2004, around 51 cases from the area had been reported, creating fear among the public.[21] Another incident during the same period was an epidemic of infective hepatitis reported from the premises of the Kottayam Medical College in the Arpookara region, where 23 cases were identified and resulted in the death of one of the medical students in the hostel.[22] The epidemic of hepatitis was traced to the inadequate biomedical waste management and drainage facilities of Kottayam Medical College's hospital. Reports of these two epidemics fuelled the already high-threat perception of fevers in the state and revived the public demand for concrete action for the control of epidemics, leading to the state's establishment of fever clinics.

In addition to the above incidents, the shift in the importance attributed to viral fever during 2003–2004 also played a role in the establishment of the fever clinics. The fear psychosis created by a sudden rise in the reported cases of dengue fever in 2003 led to a situation where even minor ailments like runny nose, sneezing, and body aches were reported as viral fever. While the elimination of private hospital reports on the grounds of biased reporting resulted in a decline in the number of dengue fever cases reported in 2004, the spotlight then shifted to the high incidence of viral fever, which led to the government's initiative to categorise it as a notifiable disease.[23] The impetus to address viral fever is evident in the following newspaper report:

> Steps have been taken for the effective control of viral fever and other infectious diseases in the State. At a meeting convened by the Health Minister, Kadavoor Sivadasan, on Monday, it was decided to start viral fever clinics at all district, taluk hospitals and major community health centres from tomorrow.[24]

Due to the heightened tendency of physicians to diagnose fevers as 'viral' along with more vigorous reporting due to its new status as a notifiable disease, the reported incidence of viral fever reached its peak in 2005 when the cases reported as well as deaths due to the disease reached double the numbers of those reported in the previous year.

In May 2004, the Kerala health ministry made the official declaration to establish fever clinics as a state-wide intervention to tackle the epidemic through surveillance and management. The characteristics and functioning were no different from those of clinics started in 2003, but extended to the whole state for the first time. Every district was to have an infectious diseases cell from which the DMOs would issue daily reports on the prevalence of viral fever and other infectious diseases. A fever register was to be maintained in all hospitals, with Rs. 800,000 sanctioned to each of the DMOs for organising activities to check viral fever. Each district was to be

---

[21]*The Hindu*, February 26, 2004.

[22]This is based on the minutes of the meetings on communicable diseases held at the DHS, Thiruvananthapuram on April 23, 2004.

[23]Minutes of the meeting on communicable diseases held on April 23, 2004, recommended the classification of viral fevers as notifiable diseases in the state.

[24]*The Hindu*, May 24, 2004.

given Rs. 74,000 for the control of dengue fever and Japanese encephalitis.[25] The circulating discourse of 'fever talk' thus resulted in the institutionalisation of fever clinics.

III

3.5 Fever Clinics at Work

According to Rosenberg, disease is:

> at once a biological event, a generation-specific repertoire of verbal constructs reflecting medicine's intellectual and institutional history, an aspect of and potential legitimation for public policy, a potentially defining element of social role, a sanction for cultural norms, and a structuring element in doctor/patient interactions. (1989: 1)

All these dimensions of viral fever as a disease were reflected in the interactions between the public health authorities, physicians, and the public in the fever clinics. In district hospitals, fever clinics were set up by providing an additional consulting room near the general medicine outpatient department (OPD), in which only patients presenting with complaints of fever were examined. The routine facilities of the general medicine department—consulting physicians, laboratory testing services, and pharmacy support—were extended to the fever clinics. The only difference was that the clinics maintained a separate record of the number of fever cases presenting to the general medicine OPD of those institutions and reported these to the authorities. A separate register was used to record the name, age, and diagnosis; however, the diagnosis was the most difficult part, so that column was usually left blank. Right from the start, many centres refused to maintain fever registers, arguing that they were already overburdened with too many tasks in the public health system. However, fever clinics did contribute to the surveillance effort by reporting fever cases to the authorities but not in the systematic manner that the latter mandated.

In the absence of a fever register, the reported number of cases was a rough estimate reached by the duty nurse, hospital attendants, and the doctor in charge of the OPD. Some hospitals estimated the number of fever patients by counting the patients who were given injections, on the assumption that those who were given injections were serious cases and possibly had viral fever. Thus, the reporting of fever was mediated by diagnostic ambiguity and the administrative inadequacies of the health services system. Despite the inadequacy of the record-keeping, the numbers generated from the PHCs, CHCs, and district hospitals and reported to the DMOs, and from there to the state-level directorate, ultimately became the data source for health planning.

---

[25]Minutes of the meetings on communicable diseases held on May 24, 2004, with the Health Minister as the convenor, also see *The Hindu* dated May 25, 2004.

3.5.1   Biomedical Practice

Following Koch's germ theory and Bernard's conception of disease as a pathological state of the body, biomedicine perceives the former as the cause and the
latter as the effect (Canguilhem 1991). Thus, disease affects the structure and
function of the body, manifested in symptoms and signs, and can be treated with
drugs (Foucault 1975). In theory, diseases are identified by the discrete sets of signs
and symptoms associated with them, as revealed by diagnostic tests categorised
within the taxonomy of biomedicine, primarily in terms of the biological characteristics of the causative agents (Brown et al. 1996). However, in actual practice,
taxonomic and diagnostic systems are based on certain cultural assumptions about
causality and normality that vary according to local traditions (ibid.). The popular
notion about biomedical practice is that it provides objective knowledge of
pathology revealed through physical findings, laboratory results, and the visual
products of contemporary imaging techniques (ibid.). In reality, it is based on the
practical reasoning and work of the physician, with the participation of the patient.

It is important to examine the roles of the physician and the patient as well as the
procedures involved in the 'medical work', to use Atkinson's term,[26] of diagnosing
and managing fevers. For Atkinson, it is these

> …socially organised practices and transactions by which facts, findings, representations,
> opinions, diagnoses—all the elements of practical medical knowledge—are produced and
> reproduced. (1995: 45)

The socialisation of physicians occurs within a dynamic medical culture
embedded in societal processes that shape physicians' perception about disease
categories. This medical culture produces what Fleck (1935) calls 'thought style'
and Friedson (2001) calls 'clinical mentality'. Given the current context of medical
practice marked by the 'pharmaceuticalisation of health' (Shiva 1985), attention
must also be paid to the role of technology and therapeutics.

3.5.2   Transactions in a Fever Clinic

A fever clinic, as a new medical institution, was usually an addendum to the
pre-existing OPDs of public hospitals ranging from CHCs to district hospitals. As is
common with government health facilities, the space for waiting was poorly fur-
nished and the majority of patients had to stand for long hours before consultation. In
the consulting room, a table was set at the centre around two chair-and-stool pairs,
arranged in such a manner that two consultations were possible whenever two

---

[26]In his study of haematologists, Atkinson (1995) analyses the activities of physicians as 'medical
work' embedded within a social and technical division of labour and grounded in material and
cultural resources.

physicians were available. On the table were instruments for checking blood pressure, a set of forms for prescribing lab tests, and medicines, mostly samples provided by medical sales representatives. The consulting room and the waiting room were separated by a screen. A stretcher in the corner of the room was occasionally used for physical examinations. Waiting patients entered the consulting room according to the order of registration, monitored by a hospital attendant.

During the consultation, doctors and patients interacted with each other and, based on the patients' responses, doctors recorded the details of the illness in a particular format in the case record. Subsequently, the patients were examined on physical parameters, the necessary laboratory tests were prescribed, and thereafter they were asked to meet the doctor with the results of the investigations. Then, the doctors prescribed medicines for a short period and asked the patient to return for a follow-up exam if required. The extent of physical examination, laboratory investigations, and prescription pattern depended upon the details of each case.

3.5.3 The Process of Diagnosis

Case 1: Rajesh, aged 32, a mason, went to the CHC. The interaction between doctor (D) and patient (P) was as follows:

D   What is your illness?
P   Severe fever and cough
D   For how long?
P   Two days
D   Do you have temperature?
P   Yes, during night the temperature is severe
D   Do you have body pain or similar symptoms?
P   During night there is severe temperature

The doctor prescribed medicine for three days and asked the patient to test his blood and urine.

The patient went home without doing the laboratory tests and was cured after taking the medicine for three days. A conversation with Rajesh at his home revealed that his leg was injured by a rock and the wound got infected, a fact that he did not mention when interacting with the doctor. The physician recorded the official diagnosis as '? PUO', indicating that the doctor suspected the illness to be pyrexia (fever) of unknown origin (PUO). According to the medical literature, the definition of PUO is elevated body temperature (> 101 °F) that lingers for at least two to three weeks and that is not due to malaria, leptospirosis, typhoid, or a range of other causes that are eliminated on the basis of intensive studies (Petersdorf 1974: 58). That is, only after ruling out a range of fevers and those fevers whose duration is more than two weeks can a diagnosis of PUO be reached. The above diagnostic process failed to follow this basic criterion. In practice, PUO becomes a convenient diagnosis when the physician does not know the reasons for presentation of fever.

Case 2: Sajitha, aged 40, a worker in the coir-manufacturing sector, came to the CHC with complaints of fever, shivering, weakness, nasal block, headache, and nausea. When she consulted the doctor for the first time, she was asked to do a sputum test, which is a common practice in that hospital as part of the tuberculosis (TB) control programme. Thereafter, she was given medicines for cough, headache, and weakness for five days. After a week, the patient returned to the hospital with the sputum test, which showed negative results for TB. The doctor then prescribed an X-ray and routine blood test, which showed high ESR.[27] After seeing the X-ray and blood report, the doctor commented: 'The lab test only shows the disease as a case of chronic obstructive pulmonary disorder (COPD), interpreted as blockage of the lung. As her husband has a history of TB and the drugs are free, it is better to treat the patient in the third category of TB patients'.[28] The doctor said this to the junior public health nurse (JPHN) who had informed the doctor that the patient's husband had suffered from TB three years ago. Treatments for cough and pulmonary obstruction were also recommended for five days. Later, when the researcher visited her home, Sajitha said that she was completely cured one week after taking the medicine for cough and pulmonary obstruction. She was quite confused about whether she should take the drugs for TB or not, as she was feeling quite well. Moreover, she pointed out that the sputum test for TB had showed negative results. The above case shows how, despite testing negative for TB, Sajitha's spouse's history of TB and the availability of drugs under the National Tuberculosis Control Programme influenced the diagnosis of a patient.

The two cases above demonstrate the process of diagnosis in 'medical work' where micro factors play a major role. In Rajesh's case, the diagnosis of suspected PUO for an illness of two days' duration contradicts the very definition of the category itself but is resorted to as a convenient diagnosis by the physician. As Fox (2000) suggests, such a categorisation is one way by which physicians manage medical uncertainties. In Sajitha's case, the physician treated her illness as TB despite the negative evidence from the sputum test and X-ray, preferring to rely on circumstantial factors and the availability of free medicines. Cases like these show that in the fever clinic the production of medical knowledge in the form of a diagnosis is not necessarily determined only by medical indications, but is based on the institutional factors, cultural assumptions, and sometimes in opposition to laboratory parameters. The search for a diagnosis is a form of active response and it is widely recognised that naming a problem offers the sufferer and his or her family

---

[27]Erythrocyte sedimentation rate (ESR) is a simple test used to determine how much inflammation is in the body, but it cannot diagnose the specific condition causing the inflammation.

[28]As the National Tuberculosis Programme was functional in that specific health centre, additional staff was provided for laboratory support for sputum examination, along with free medicines for TB.

a degree of control through certainty that must itself be considered therapeutic (Samson 1999). Yet, in the cases described above, the diagnoses did not generate any such therapeutic effect.

IV

3.6   Discourses on Institutionalising an Epidemic

Disease-specific studies in an Indian context unravel the multiple interpretations of an event and have an important contribution to the response of the actors, including the state. Addlakha (2001), in her study on the dengue epidemic in Delhi during 1996, also examined how the state, the media, the medical fraternity, and the individual citizen responded during an epidemic in the National Capital Region (NCR). Using a multi-sited ethnography, she demonstrated how an epidemic is dealt with as a crisis by the prevalent structures, and in the process, how selective silencing and erasures happen at different levels, where the power of the legal apparatus legitimises state interventions, thereby maintaining the stability of the state.

This chapter examined the journey of 'fever' from symptom to epidemic in Kerala. Though the category of 'fevers' has been always prevalent in society, its meaning has changed extensively over time. The use of the 'exclusionary principle' in diagnosing fevers led to large-scale attribution of these illnesses as 'viral fevers'. During the mid-1990s, fevers were recognised as an 'epidemic'; cases of fever—especially fatal ones—were highlighted by the media to create a circulating discourse of 'fever talk'; the government was prompted to take the initiative by establishing fever clinics. The techniques of surveillance and reporting in the fever clinics, though quite haphazard, further contributed to the production of knowledge about fevers as an epidemic. It is obvious how this notion of fevers as an epidemic emerged with the significant support of biomedicine, the dominant system of medicine prevalent. This development is incongruous, as biomedical understanding authorises fever only as an elevated body temperature that ought to be treated as a symptom. The contradiction within biomedicine is further heightened in the fever clinics, where the basic diagnostic categories used and the knowledge that guides clinical practice both diverge from theoretical biomedical knowledge. Rather, it is the social and institutional micro factors within clinical practice that determine diagnosis. In this process of institutionalisation, alternative approaches to understanding and managing fevers cast aside.

References

Addlakha, R. (2001). State legitimacy and social suffering in a modern epidemic: A case study of dengue haemorrhagic fever in Delhi. *Contributions to Indian Sociology, 35*(2), 151–179.

Atkinson, P. (1995). *Medical talk and medical work: The liturgy of the clinic.* London: Sage Publications.

Banerji, D. (1984). Breakdown of public health system. *Economic and Political Weekly, 19*(22), 881–882.

Brown, P. J., Inhorn, M. C., & Smith, D. J. (1996). Disease, ecology and human behaviour. In C. F. Sargent & T. M. Johnson (Eds.), *Medical anthropology: Contemporary theory and method* (Revised edition ed., pp. 183–219). Connecticut, London: Praeger.

Canguilhem, G. (1991). *On the normal and the pathological.* New York: Zone Books.

Fleck, L. (1981 [1935]). On the question of the foundation of medical knowledge. *Journal of Medicine and Philosophy, 6* (3), 237–256.

Foucault, M. (1975). *The birth of the clinic: Archaeology of medical perception.* New York and London: Vintage Books.

Fox, R. C. (2000). Medical uncertainty revisited. In L. A. Gary, R. Fitzptrick, & S. C. Scrimshaw (Eds.), *Handbook of social studies in health and medicine,* London: Sage.

Fox, R. C. (1957). Training for uncertainty. In R. K. Merton, G. G. Reader & P. L. Kendall (Eds.), *The student physician* (pp. 204–241). Cambridge, MA: Harvard University Press.

Friedson, E. (2001 [1970]). The profession of medicine. In M. Purdy & D. Banks (Eds.), *The sociology and politics of health: A reader* (pp. 130–134). London: Routledge.

George, M. (2007a). *Interpreting fever talk and fever care in Kerala's socio-cultural context* (Unpublished Ph D thesis). Centre of Social Medicine and Community Health, School of Social Sciences, Jawaharlal Nehru University, New Delhi.

George, M. (2007b). Socio–Economic and cultural dimensions and health seeking behaviour for leptospirosis: A case study of Kerala. *Journal of Health Management, 9*(3), 381–398.

Jorgensen, M., & Phillips, L. (2002). *Discourse analysis as theory and method.* London: Sage.

Kannan, K. P., Thankappan, K. R., Ramankutty, V., & Aravindan, K. P. (1991). *Health and development in rural Kerala.* Thiruvananthapuram, Kerala: Kerala Sastra Sahithya Parishad.

Kohl, K. S., Marcy, M., Blum, M., Jones, M. C., Dagan, R., Hansen, J., et al. (2004). Fever after immunization: Current concepts and improved future scientific understanding. *Clinical Infectious Diseases, 39*(3), 389–394.

Krishnaswami, P. (2004). *Morbidity study—Incidence, prevalence, consequences and associates,* Discussion Paper No. 63, Thiruvananthapuram: Kerala Research Programme on Local Level Development, Centre for Development Studies.

Kunjhikannan, T. P., & Aravindan, K. P. (2000). *Changes in health transition in Kerala, 1987–1997.* Thiruvananthapuram: Kerala Research Programme on Local Level Development, Centre for Development Studies.

Mackowaik, P. A. (1998, September 28). Concepts of fever, *Archives of Internal Medicine. 158* (17), 1870–1881.

Mackowiak, P. A., Bartlett, J., Borden, E. C., Goldblum, S. E., Hasday, J. D., Munford, R. S., et al. (1997). Concepts of fever: Recent advances and lingering dogma. *Clinical Infectious Diseases, 25*(1), 119–138.

Naraindas, H. (2006). Of spineless babies and folic acid: Evidence and efficacy in biomedicine and ayurvedic medicine. *Social Science and Medicine, 62*(11), 2658–2669.

Panicker, P. G. K., & Soman, C. R. (1984). *Health status of Kerala: The paradox of economic backwardness and health development.* Thiruvananthapuram, Kerala: Centre for Development Studies.

Petersdorf, R. G. (1974). Disturbances of heat regulation. In M. M. Wintrobe, G. W. Thorn, R. D Adams, E. Braunwald, K. J Isselbacher, & R. G. Petersdorf (Eds.), Harrison's principles of internal medicine (7th ed., pp. 48–62). New Delhi: Tata McGraw Hill.

Ramachandran, R. (2006, October 07–20). Virulent Outbreak. *Frontline, 23*(20). Available at http://www.frontlineonnet.com/fl2320/stories/20061020004911900.htm. Accessed on May 22, 2010.

Remadevi, S., & Dass, S. (1999). *Environmental factors of malaria persistence: A study at Valiyathura, Thiruvananthapuram City*. Discussion Paper No. 3, Thiruvananthapuram: Kerala Research Programme on Local Level Development, Centre for Development Studies.

Samson, C. (1999). The physician and the patient. In C. Samson (Ed.), *Health studies, A critical and cross cultural reader*. United Kingdom: Blackwell Publishers.

Shiva, M. (1985). Towards a healthy use of pharmaceuticals: An Indian perspective. *Development Dialogue, 2*, 69–93.

Yardley, L. (Ed.). (1997). *Material discourses of health and illness*. London: Routledge.

Chapter 4
Fear of Fevers: Risk, Medicalisation, and Provisioning

Abstract This chapter examines how the societal discourse on fevers interferes with people's perceptions and health-seeking behaviours. This is accomplished by interpreting various notions about fever as understood by those affected with the illness during and after experiencing the illness, along with examining the diverse practices followed by people for 'managing' fevers. The meanings attributed to fever by the public reveal that the lay understanding is tuned both by one's way of life as well as by what has emanated from the dominant biomedical understanding. These varied notions of fever can be seen as an interaction of multiple knowledge systems prevalent in the society, and they are at times in mutual conflict or in concordance. This is contextualised within the sociocultural context of contemporary Kerala society, which reports increased rates of caesarian section, greater antibiotic use, and greater acceptance and use of high-end medical technology, all indicating a highly consumerist state even for medical care. Further, in a society grappling with the fear of an illness, emerging from the 'perceived' risk of death results in a medicalised society, and raising the 'standard' of medical care by offering quality services then becomes the need of the hour as projected by the private health care facilities. Thus, there is a risk-driven medicalised society that raises the 'standard' for medical care, and whose needs are 'satisfied' by the dominant private-sector health care through its provisioning. This is a reciprocal process, as higher standards of medical care lead to further medicalisation and rising aspirations of consumers for medical care.

Keywords Risk and medicalisation · Provisioning of medical care · Commercialisation in fever care · Burden of fevers

4.1 Introduction

This chapter examines how the societal discourse on fevers interferes with people's perceptions and health seeking behaviours. This is accomplished by interpreting various notions about fever as understood by those affected with the illness during and after experiencing the illness, along with examining the diverse practices followed by people for 'managing' fevers. This is contextualised within the socio-cultural context of contemporary Kerala wherein the acceptance of the latest medical procedures is higher than in other Indian states, and has also resulted in what economists have characterised as 'mediflation', where the 'value' of medicine and medical care has been reduced due to greater supply (Kunjhikannan and Aravindan 2000). Moreover, studies of the state of Kerala, traditionally known for its paradox of higher morbidity with good health indicators—especially lower mortality indicators—have attributed its population's greater health consciousness as leading to higher rates of self-reported morbidities, which Sen (2002) attributes to a 'perception factor'. The recent development of increased caesarian section rates (Thankappan 2001), greater antibiotic use (Saradama et al. 2000), and greater acceptance and use of high-end medical technology within the state all need to be seen as an indication of a highly consumerist state, even for medical care, which some scholars have cautioned to the possibility of Kerala following a US model of commercialised health care (Ekbal 2000). It is in this context, the following questions will be addressed in this chapter. What are the ways in which patients and health care facilities interpret fevers? How do patients understand the cause, cure, care, and 'risk' regarding fevers? What financial and other difficulties (burdens) have patients had to face due to the illness? What is the health-seeking behaviour of patients affected with fever?

This chapter uses the results of interviews of fever patients identified and selected from four different hospitals where they sought care for fevers, and from subsequent follow-up using a survey technique with these patients at their homes after being cured of the illness one month later. The hospitals selected included two public and two private-sector hospitals that offer primary- and secondary-level care from one of the municipal corporations (city areas). Within the private sector, Sivani hospital, a small hospital rendering primary-level care, and Immanuel hospital, which renders secondary level care, were selected (the names of the hospitals have been changed to ensure anonymity). The details of each hospital and their infrastructure facilities are already mentioned in Chap. 1. Fever patients were identified from the hospitals where patients received treatment, as data shows that in the state of Kerala, around 90 % of those having any illness seek treatment in some type of health facility (NSSO 1998: A-40 & A-145). It was also found that among those who seek treatment, around 80 % are treated in the allopathic system for acute illnesses (Aravindan 2006). Thus, an allopathic hospital-based study of fevers in Kerala can ensure more than 72 %[1] coverage of the total fever patients in the community. Recent surveys have shown that utilisation of the allopathic system among Kerala has increased to around 90 % (NSSO 2014).

---

[1]In this community, of the 90 % of patients who reach a hospital in case of illness, 80 % go to an allopathic hospital. Based on this information, it can be deduced that 72 % (90 × 80 % = 72) of those with acute illness seek treatment at allopathic hospitals.

4.2   Selection of Patients

Those patients presenting to the OPD for the first time with perceived fever, with symptoms of headache, elevated body temperature, body pain, nausea, etc., and whose fever was not due to early infections like TB, asthma, and other chronic diseases met the criteria of fever patients for the study. As the study confines itself only to fever patients, 40 fever patients were selected from the OPDs of each hospital, together making a final sample of 160 patients from four different hospitals. This was carried out by dividing the total outpatient time of each hospital into four phases and randomly picking up a specific number of cases (based on the patient load) from each phase. The patient's consent and their contact address for follow-up were collected while they were on the hospital premises.

Those patients identified and selected at the hospitals were followed to their respective homes, and a detailed study on their understanding and perceptions about health, illness, cure, and care was carried out. The survey captured how the patients responded to fever at the time of ill health (their health-seeking behaviour) and the difficulties faced, as well as their understanding of fever with respect to its cause, possible cure, and available treatment facilities. This afforded a better understanding of the differences in the burden of fevers across social groups, as well as the difference in the nature of care rendered by different health facilities.

4.3   Health-Seeking Behaviour

The concept of *health-seeking behaviour,* which takes into account the role of social structures in the behaviour of patients, will be elaborated here. The concept of health-seeking behaviour is not dealt with uniformly, as some authors consider it synonymous with treatment-seeking behaviour (Ward et al. 1997). Here, health-seeking behaviour is interpreted as those behaviours that directly or indirectly contribute to health both at the time of illness and during its absence. This broader conceptualisation not only incorporates the role of social structures in human behaviour but also enables an examination of a person's understanding and perception of health and illness as a product of constant interaction with the prevalent structures. Unlike the health belief model, perception and understanding of health and illness are seen here as an outcome of people's past experiences with their illness and their engagement with the prevalent social institutions to deal with it.

Health-seeking behaviour incorporates health behaviour, illness behaviour, and treatment-seeking behaviour. *Health behaviours* are those behaviours knowingly or unknowingly performed in an asymptomatic (no illness) stage as part of the life that can retain health (Steele and McBroom 1972). These include behaviours carried out to retain health while a person is in a healthy state, like those provided by the health services for health promotion, such as vaccinations. Along with it, behaviours like drinking safe water and following better sanitary facilities can be included in this category. This concept can be used to invoke the need for adequate food, safe working conditions, basic housing facilities, safe water supply, and sanitation in a society that ultimately becomes the prerequisite for ensuring better health behaviour. The above concept of health behaviour will depend on people's notions about their health (wellbeing), as their health behaviour is a function of the latter.

Illness behaviours as defined by Mechanic (1969: 191) *are the ways in which given symptoms are perceived, evaluated, and acted (or not acted) upon by different people.* In other words, it is the way by which illness (un-wellness) is expressed by people. The social context within illness behaviour is strongly asserted by Alonzo (1984) who addresses how various situations of everyday life can suppress certain illness behaviours among certain groups, whereas for others, the same illness will become a serious concern. The need to examine social structures, including social networks, in the perception of health and illness is further emphasised by Suchman (1963) and recently by Mechanic (1993). The latter, also a proponent of illness behaviour, was approached by physicians to study it for each disease for the purpose of better diagnosis, as illness behaviour was broadly considered by physicians to be similar to symptoms and thus treated as an individual psychological entity. The earlier concept of illness was premised on the understanding of disease as a physiological entity and illness as a sociological one, attributing a taken-for-granted status to disease. The statement, 'It is quite possible to be ill without being diseased, and also can [sic] have disease without being ill', best reveals the contextual relevance of illness behaviour (Loustaunau and Sobo 1997: 87). As is obvious from the illness/disease debates, illness is not merely a person's reaction to a disease but his/her experience of suffering, which differs from the medical category of *disease.* Therefore, past experiences (direct or indirect) of the patient with the type of suffering can influence the way he/she behaves. This is because illness behaviour is very much linked to the patient's understanding of the cause of the distress, their understanding of what is *normal,* and also the *visibility* and frequency of the symptom (Loustaunau and Sobo 1997: 87). This understanding (meaning) about the symptoms and their characteristics in turn could be an outcome of the dominant prevailing knowledge as well as the type of knowledge generated by the social institutions, especially health care facilities. Thus, a dominant position for disease fails to strengthen the concept of illness behaviour, which can otherwise be a potential tool embedded in context and made relevant for social research in public health.

Lastly, the concept of treatment-seeking behaviour is defined as that part of illness behaviour extending to seeking treatment—those activities undertaken by individuals who perceive themselves as having a health problem or as being ill, and who desire to be rid of the illness. Treatment-seeking behaviour, like the earlier two concepts, is also dependent on prevalent social structures, especially the available medical care facilities. Mere availability of medical care does not ensure access to services, as the available services should cater to the social, cultural, and more importantly, economic needs of the people (Sagar 1994). It is in this context that treatment-seeking behaviour at one level has the power to question the provisioning of medical care by sectors in terms of its adequacy, responsiveness, and quality. In other words, those factors influencing the utilisation of health services in general, and medical care in particular, from a people-centric perspective can be understood using the concept of treatment-seeking behaviour.

4.4 Interpreting Fevers in Kerala

Using the above concepts of health-seeking behaviour, this section examines fever patients and their understanding about the illness (fever) they suffer from. This will be examined both during the advancement of illness, i.e. illness behaviour of the patient, and after getting relief from the illness together with their perceived causes of fever and their source of knowledge. This is the period during which a patient perceives his/her illness until the patient reaches any health facility. For Suchman (1963), the *symptom experience* stage and *assumption of sick role* stage together constitute illness behaviour. Using this perspective and applying it to *fevers* (a patient-centric sociological category that encompasses a range of illness), an in-depth analysis of *illness behaviour* is attempted. It is worth mentioning here that *fevers* as an illness category renders different meanings for different people.

4.4.1 Fever as that Which Interrupts Day-to-Day Life

In the earlier chapter on the contemporary discourses on fever, it was demonstrated that this discourse was more inclined towards biomedical understanding, the dominant and widely utilised system of medicine in the state. Similar to the case of other illnesses, fever is understood in diverse ways, especially as it is perceived as a hindrance to normal life. This was reflected in using the term *pani* (fever) for *kshinam* (fatigue), *thalarcha* (weakness: especially unable to do anything), and sometimes a more direct usage of *joley cheyyan pattunnilla* [unable to work (daily)].

The linkage between fever and body heat was obvious during clinical interactions reflected in a physician's counter-question, 'whether there is *choodu*' (temperature/heat), when patients complained of *pani* (fever). It has to be noted that *choodu* (meaning heat) is also used in Kerala society to express profuse sweating of the body due to excess humidity. This dual meaning of *choodu* at times resulted in doctors' misinterpreting it as *body heat*, when the patients actually meant profuse sweating. Another perceived cause of *pani* (fever) is mental stress, which people attribute to anger, jealousy, and so on, that can also lead to illness—for which *pani* is the term used. This lay perception can be considered logical given that some scholars have also identified usage of the term *choodu* to indicate a strong heat due to anger or jealousy, for example, which is negatively valued by society (Osella and Osella 1996).

4.4.2 Tracing the Causes

Further, patients' perceived cause(s) of fever were examined and the results indicated that around 22 % consider *climate* as an important factor, for 18 % it was *bathing habits,* and 11 % consider *hard labour* as the cause of fever. It is worth mentioning here that 37 % of the studied population said that they *do not know* the cause of fever. Upon further analysis with respect to the occupation of the patient, it was found that the daily-wage labourer was the major group represented among respondents, and considered *hard labour* and *climate* as the causes of fever. For the student community, factors such as bathing habits, climate, and an unsafe environment were perceived as the causes of fever. In other words, illness itself was perceived to be more of an outcome of their *way of life* for each group of patients rather than due to *microbes.* The sources of the above knowledge reassert this argument, as a majority (42.4 %) identified past experience with similar illness and its care as the main source of understanding about the illness. In other words, those affected with illness perceive it mostly as being caused due to the alterations in their normal way of life, and this understanding is restructured and reshaped by their direct and indirect experiences with similar illnesses and their engagement with health care facilities. This is very similar to the cultural epidemiological approach of explaining illness from patients' perspectives, which according to the emic approach is an outcome of the pattern of distress (PD) interpreted based on their perceived causes, and which in turn triggers their help-seeking behaviour (Weiss 2001).

Upon tracing the term *pani,* the literal meaning in the vernacular dictionary was found to be *dew, cool,* whereas the popular meaning has been *an illness with elevated body temperature,* the latter owing to the biomedical explanation. The earlier two explanations, when examined with the causes of fever as reported by the patients like *climatic conditions* as well as *bathing habits,* show strong linkages. It should be noted that the causes of fever identified by patients raise the possibility of an alternative understanding of fever (*pani*) that still exists in the society.

In short, the understanding of fever can be explained as a combination of diverse perspectives. First, there is a traditional notion of *fever* (*pani*) as something that has to do with climate owing to the literal meaning of *dew* and *cool.* Second, the reasons for attributing the causes of fever as being due to *problems in bathing habits* (unhealthy ways of cooling the body) could be traced to the meaning of *pani* as *cool.* This is revealed from the statements of patients who attribute *bathing immediately after hard labour* or after *excessive travel* to be the cause of fever. Finally, the notion of fever (*pani*) as elevated body temperature runny nose, and common cold could be based on socialisation from biomedicine, as it is close to the biomedical understanding of fever. It is worth mentioning here that the latter interpretation of fever as that of raised body temperature, runny nose, and common cold is largely used and propagated by a majority of patients and their relatives. Factors such as climate and bathing habits pop up only during informal conversation is initiated, and especially at their home setting as opposed to in a hospital setting. Only for the purpose of explanation can these be differentiated, as many of these notions can overlap and can supplement one another.

It should also be noted that the illness behaviour at one level reveals the prevalent discourse on fever, where the influence of a disease threat is obvious. Illness behaviour when linked to a patient's way of life—especially to the daily wage labourer—calls for the need to ensure basic working and living conditions that become a prerequisite for better health behaviours. Additionally, it is necessary to note that the varied notions of fever that are prevalent in the society are rational and can be traced to the lineage of the term, which has a bearing on the socio-cultural context of the society. Here, it is interesting that diverse meanings that still exist within the society for a simple illness like fever, of which the dominant understanding comes from biomedicine, potentially due to its dominance.

4.4.3 Fever: During and After Suffering

In order to understand the change in individuals' perceptions of fevers during different phases of illness, an attempt was made to understand patient perceptions during and after the illness. This is based on the understanding that the power of experience in making sense of an event is more significant and long-standing than the way in which it is understood through hearsay. This is also considered an additional benefit of an anthropologist's inquiry of an illness over that of an epidemiological inquiry, where the former situates 'experience' at the centre of meaning creation (Trostle 2005). Those patients affected with fevers were asked within a month after being cured to reflect on how they felt while suffering from their illness. It was interesting to see that a large majority of the patients considered their fever mostly as a symptom, while some perceived it as a disease and only a few perceived it as an 'epidemic'. A few others preferred to situate it somewhere between a symptom and a disease. Here, the assumption was that a symptom meant the less severe kind of fever and an epidemic the most severe, with disease in between along a continuum. This pattern indicates the ambiguity around the idea of fever as it exists in a society where a large proportion perceives it as a symptom, possibly influenced by the outcome of the dominant biomedical understanding. Those who consider fever either as a disease or as an epidemic demonstrate that there is an influence of fever threat (fear) in the state. Those who want to situate fever somewhere between a symptom and a disease represent the voices of dissent toward the dominant categories who are thereby trying to understand the problem differently.

Moreover, based on the cases followed, it was found that at the time of suffering at the hospital patients themselves felt that their fever was serious and needed some immediate attention. Once the illness subsided, many of them shared the feeling that their illness was very mild, using terms like *normal, simple fevers,* and *simple cold-related fevers,* and recovered in two to three days, sometimes with medication and other times without. It was interesting to find that the notion of fever threat was built up slowly and then got diffused, mostly triggered by pressure from the immediate relatives of the patients: parents in the case of the unmarried, spouses in case of the married (25–40 age group), and also sons/daughters pressuring their older (50+) parents. In short, the decision for seeking treatment is so complex that one has to go beyond the institutional factors as well as the *doctor characteristics* for a better understanding.

This becomes obvious when one examines the purpose for which a patient consults a doctor at the time of illness. There are patients who demand specific tablets for their illnesses based on their earlier experiences. Some demand laboratory tests to rule out their perceived threat of certain epidemics or diseases, whereas others demand admittance to the hospital even against the doctor's will. In short, the purposes of patients coming to the hospital for consultation of fever vary widely, reflected in the presentation of their illness to the physician. In other words, the perception of fevers by the patient is mediated by the prevalent threat of a societal epidemic, triggered by an understanding of being at 'risk', along with the better availability of health care facilities in a society that is highly consumerist.

4.5   Biomedical Interpretation of *Fevers*

The biomedical interpretation of fever was based on information about fever patients who sought treatment from four different hospitals in the state. The purpose was to situate people's interpretations of fever as there is a popular notion that hospital-based classification is more '*scientific*' and reliable, as it is closer to reality. Per the survey, it was astonishing to find that only 14 % (21) of the total sample ($N = 151$) had a confirmed diagnosis, 22 % (33) had a suspected diagnosis, and the rest [64 % (97)] were categorised only up to the symptom level. This not only resulted in an inability to use the final valid diagnosis as an indicator to understand the illness but also a limit to understanding the severity of the prevalent types of fevers. Further, among those with a final diagnosis (14 %) of acute respiratory infection (ARI), lower and upper respiratory tract infections constituted the majority of cases, with some reported as having viral fever with two cases of pyrexia of unknown origin (PUO). The above cases further indicate that even those fevers that reached hospitals and had final diagnoses do not report serious illnesses that need to be feared, as there was not even a single case that fell into the category of 'epidemic' fevers. In addition, among those with a suspected diagnosis (22 %), it was found that those with viral fever were in the highest proportion, with acute respiratory infection (ARI) ranking next. Further, as most of the patients were diagnosed only up to the symptom level (43.7 %), it indicates that a good proportion of fever patients presenting at health facilities in Kerala society are those with common illnesses that are possibly not very serious. This has been the characteristic of other

Table 4.1 Severe symptoms of the patients (self-perceived) and their mean duration of illness

Severe symptoms	No. of patients	Percentage	Mean duration of *fever* (illness)	Mean duration for seeking treatment
Rise in temperature	29	19.2	9.07	2.62
Body pain/back pain	28	18.5	13.46	3.36
Cough/throat pain	23	15.2	11.43	3.61
Accumulation of Phlegm	19	12.6	7.74	2.79
Headache	17	11.3	8.06	2.76
Rash	14	9.3	10.00	2.50
Breathing difficulty	7	4.6	11.14	4.00
Sneezing	6	4.0	7.00	3.17
Joint pain	3	2.0	13.67	5.33
Others	5	3.3	13.80	2.40
Total	151	100.0	10.31	3.25

Source Author

societies as well as in Kerala during all periods where *fevers of short duration* have been a significant category, as revealed by several surveys (NSSO 1998; Kannan et al. 1991; Kunjhikannan and Aravindan 2000).

In short, it was obvious that most of the fevers that were treated at various hospitals in the contemporary period were neither severe nor indicative of any specific 'epidemic' fevers. Therefore, even a biomedical interpretation of fevers does not justify society's fear of them as an 'epidemic' or as a 'disease'. Despite this, there are risk perceptions about fevers among the community that also contribute to the overall fever discourse in the state. This became obvious when data about the most severe symptoms and the total duration of fevers was examined for 151 patients who sought treatment from four different hospitals of the state. Table 4.1 shows the most severe symptom reported by patients, the total duration of treatment, and the mean duration of the illness.

From Table 4.1, it is clear that the mean duration for one episode of fever was around 10 days. For those with severe symptoms of back pain and joint pain, the mean duration of illness was around 13 days, and for those with breathing difficulty and throat pain/cough, the mean duration was around 11 days. Those who complained of rashes and a rise in temperature as their severe symptoms had a mean duration of 10 and 9 days, respectively. The pattern of severe symptoms and the mean duration of illness further confirm that the majority of the illnesses studied were not very serious, as the duration ranged from one to two weeks, a characteristic of minor fevers.

4.6 Lay Versus Medical Categorisation

The lay and medical interpretations of *fevers* not only illustrate the variations in prevalent conceptions about fevers in the society but also provide an impression of the nature and characteristics of the fevers with respect to their severity. A comparison between the interpretations of fever by the people as well as by the medical fraternity reveals whether these interpretations are in agreement or in conflict. A clear distinction is obvious between the perceptions of fever as understood by lay people and by the biomedical interpretation. For lay people, illness is understood more as that which hinders their daily life in terms their 'natural' ability to do work, which reasserts the earlier argument that people understand diseases through their lived experiences rather than the presence or absence of microbes or symptoms (Trostle 2005). However, in terms of severity it is important to note that despite a different interpretation of the event, there has been a convergence wherein both the public and the field of biomedicine agreed that the type of illness were not very severe, the former based upon an experiential logic and the latter from a 'scientific' logic. The above pattern clearly reveals that there exists a commonality between the medical interpretation and the public's interpretation of fevers in terms of illness severity, though they might have articulated 'fevers' differently according to their 'thought style'.

Ghosh and Coutinho (2000) in their study on cholera in Kolkata during 1994–1995 found that the understanding by the medical fraternity and the public about cholera was widely varied, where the former understood the disease as mostly due to a change in the strain of the virus and therefore having increased *infectivity*. For the latter, the disease was perceived more as a lived experience where the crisis was mostly in terms of the people's inability to lead a *normal* life. The problem becomes more serious when it was found that similar to any other infections, the majority of those affected belonged to the lower socio-economic group, which also led to *victim blaming*, another common strategy of escapism by the state from civic responsibility. Victim blaming is identified not merely as a cornering of the deprived but more importantly as how the construction of the *self* and *other* gets accomplished through this process. Moreover, it is noteworthy that living conditions constrained the health-seeking behaviour of those affected and, despite the prevalence of biomedicine, how the *quacks* and other healers played a significant role in providing care to the slum dwellers. Another study by Prasad (2005) on malaria in Gujarat during the period 1995–2000 examined the human factors that social scientific research highlights or undermines as the processes in the identification of malaria, its causes, and subsequent treatment process. He argues that there exists a strong distinction between the *lay* and *expert* perception of malaria as a disease, thereby representing two different realities rather than a shared *reality*. Not only is this distinction in understanding found in the case of sickness but also is true for its cause as well as its cure.

4.6.1 Perceiving Fevers

The above section clearly reveals that multiple discourses about fever exist within Kerala society. Broadly, one may categorise these into the public's perspective and an expert or a biomedical perspective. There are further differences within the public's perspective depending on their thought style and acts of engagement. Here, the close association of fevers with people's lived experience is an important characteristic that is demonstrated from an anthropological perspective. Furthermore, the diversity in understanding also reveals the multiplicity of human engagement with an event, thus creating possibilities for change. However, the dominant biomedical understanding and the power it has on the lay public's understanding is also a reality. What is more important is that the threat generated within a society about epidemics in general and fever epidemics in particular, and the power of that threat to shape and reshape the understanding of an illness, is an area needing greater attention. There is a thin line between the perception of fear and that of risk, as the former is often treated as an impulsive response without necessarily an explanation or evidence, whereas in the case of risk, there is gen-erally assumed to be a logical reason premised on existing evidence that channels the perception of risk.

This opens up the need to understand the discourse on risk in the field of public health and its implications. Scholars who have worked on risk discourse in this context have elaborated that risk originally was only viewed as a probability for any event (positive or negative), but has eventually transformed to that of a probability of the occurrence of danger and hence is seen predominantly in a negative light (Lupton 1993; Rothstein 2003). Fox (1999) further elaborates that mere risk esti-mation is not enough, since for every event it is possible to calculate a statistically probable risk for a range of factors. In reality, whether this risk actually translates into danger depends upon the contextual nature in which the society and the events are constituted. In other words, the very notion of something being at risk is based on the societal knowledge about what counts as evidence, hazard, and likelihood of an event and so on, all of which are always constructed in a given society and viewed from a given standpoint. Unlike the traditional form in which a previous experience of hazard was the starting point for risk assessment, in the contemporary context it is the risk assessment that projects a future hazard, wherein the latter exists only through the projection of the former, further creating a subjective per-ception of risk among people that, according to Fox (1999), is a form of postmodern reflection on risk.

When this is examined in the context of fevers in Kerala society, it is important to note that the institutions of fever clinics and the media together create a scenario wherein there is a subjective risk perception among people about fevers. What is the actual hazard in this context? It could be the possibility of those fevers becoming any of the 'epidemic fevers[2]', which if not treated in time can be fatal. If we consider the probability of an individual suffering from the hazard of any epidemic fevers among the total number of those affected with fevers, it is certain to be considerably less, as only very few cases among the large number of fever cases reported in hospitals are epidemic fevers. The hazards of epidemic fevers in the state are far less than is projected, and mostly confined to areas that are endemic to leptospirosis and malaria. This brings us to consider the possibility that a significant level of epidemic fever hazard does not exist in actuality, but only (virtually) through the estimation of risk based on the subjective perception of fever threat among the public. Similar situations exist in the field of public health, where risk assessment becomes the origin and is attributed as the cause of virtual hazard, wherein the actual hazard is much less than that which is prospectively projected. The case of the rotavirus vaccine for preventing diarrhoeal disorders and exclusive health insurance for inpatients as a way of reducing catastrophic expenditures were both based on the posing of a virtual hazard (based on risk estimation) at a higher level than the actual occurrence of the hazard in reality. The rotavirus vaccine is promoted as a solution to diarrhoeal diseases among children, when in reality, the population data shows that less than 30 % of all diarrhoeal diseases are caused by various strains of the rotavirus. The case of health insurance schemes is similar, which in India is exclusively for hospitalisation: though only 5–10 % of the population need hospitalisation annually, 100 % coverage of health insurance is promoted as a way to avoid catastrophic health expenditures. In both of the above cases, it is the 'individual risk' involved in the event that is projected more aggressively, and addressing it is viewed as a solution to preventing the 'hazard'. This has resulted in serious policy debates within the field of health policy on questions of prioritisation. These risks and therefore the hazards can be justified only if, in the case of vaccination, the population data show significantly high incidence rates of the diseases under consideration for prevention, in the case of health insurance and a very high rate of hospitalisation in a population.

---

[2]Epidemic fevers are those diseases with fever as major symptoms that struck in epidemic proportions and created havoc in the state by the middle of the 1990s, marked by greater fatality and being new and unfamiliar to common people. They include Japanese encephalitis reported during 1996–1998, and leptospirosis, popularly known as rat fever and which doctors claim to have treated since the 1980s, reported in epidemic proportions since 1998 and continuing until the present (although the death due to this disease has reduced since 2002). Subsequently, dengue fever showed its face in 2001 with its peak during 2003, and gradually declined from the next year on when viral fever became the new culprit, which attained its peak in 2005 and 2006. The culmination was in the epidemic of chikungunya fever in July 2006 when there was a huge controversy on the disease per se and the cause of deaths during the period.

4.6.2 *Response to Fevers*

It is important to examine the ways that people respond to fevers in terms of seeking care, which include those activities people engage in to get rid of the illness. The concept of treatment-seeking behaviour will help to clarify these sets of activities. Treatment-seeking behaviour is defined as those activities undertaken by individuals who perceive themselves as having a health problem or being ill, in order to get rid of the illness. As mentioned earlier, Suchman's (1963) *stages of illness experience* that comprise the stages of *medical care contact, dependent patient role,* and *recovery or rehabilitation,* together constitute treatment-seeking behaviour. Scholars have identified that immediately after recognising (perceiving) the illness, patients usually try home remedies as well as self-medication and various other behaviours before utilising any health facility to get rid of the illness (Sushama 1990). Before entering into a discussion of contemporary treatment-seeking behaviour, a brief account of the ways by which fevers were managed during 1960s and 1970s in the state is worth mentioning, as it can help to explain the current trend.

Despite the dominance of modern medicine by the mid-twentieth century, a range of home remedies was used in Kerala to manage fevers. These included intake of black coffee mixed with pepper and *chukku* (dried ginger), taking *kanji* (rice porridge) and *kurumulakurasam* (pepper soup), and an array of other preparations. Only if this failed did people go to local practitioners and finally to the allopathic system (Ramachandran 2000). In other words, it is obvious that fever as an illness was managed effectively in homes in Kerala society during the 1960s. It should be noted that Kerala was free of malaria by the mid-1960s, which led to a situation where fever was never a threat for the people until the 1990s when it struck hard as an epidemic. In the present study, attempts were made to understand the behaviours of the patients during their experience of this illness. It was found that *steam-inhalation*[3] as well as *kashayam* (a preparation similar to black coffee with jaggery, black pepper, and ginger as ingredients) taken during fever were the two major home remedies practised. It was also found that even in the contemporary period, those who tried home remedies—which is still a significant proportion—tried either steam-inhalation or *kashayam,* and a few had tried both. On being asked the reasons for this, one woman replied, 'earlier this had been enough, but now this is not safe, as there are new varieties of fever and also there are deaths due to fevers'. This divulges not only the usefulness of home remedies in the past but also the replacement of these practices by others. The reasons could be the changing nature of fevers and the prevalent perception of their threat to wellbeing, as well as greater access to health services.

---

[3]Steam inhalation is a procedure carried out by subjecting the patient's head and at times the upper part of the body to steam. The steam is made by boiling plain water, and—usually for medicinal value—a range of products from Eucalyptus or Vicks balm, and so on, will be mixed with the boiling water. For the procedure to be more effective, the body and the boiled water are covered with a blanket, allowing the body to sweat profusely.

Table 4.2 Patients who tried home remedies versus self-medication

Whether self-medicated	Any home remedies		Total
	Yes	No	
Yes	12 (34.29) [26.1]	23 (65.71) [21.9]	35 (100) [23.2]
No	34 (29.31) [73.9]	82 (70.69) [78.1]	116 (100) [76.8]
Total	46 (30.46) [100.0]	105 (69.54) [100.0]	151 (100.0) [100.0]

Source Primary survey, 2007
Note () denotes row percentage and [ ] denotes column percentage

Additionally, some patients reported trying self-medication, which constitutes buying medicines directly from the chemist and consuming them during illness without a valid prescription from the doctor. The amazing fact is that almost all patients who bought medicines without a valid prescription opted for paracetamol or its derivative. In order to understand the transition in the treatment-seeking pattern of patients with fevers, two specific behaviours related to fevers where observed. As part of the data generated through the survey, comparisons were made between patients who had followed home remedies and self-medication.

Table 4.2 shows that only 46 patients (30.46 %) tried home remedies before going to a health facility, whereas those who self-medicated totalled 35 (23.2 %). It should be noted that those who had taken home remedies as well as medicated themselves had later gone to some health facility. The interesting part is that among those who tried home remedies, a majority (74 %) of them had not tried self-medication, and a significant (66 %) majority of those who tried self-medication had not tried home remedies. If medicalisation is seen as a process and self-medication as an indication of it, then it can be argued that those who tried home remedies alone have not yet entered into the stages of medicalisation, whereas those who undertake self-medication alone are more medicalised. In other words, the former group is less medicalised than the latter. Thus, one can argue that in the state of Kerala self-medication practices might have replaced those home remedies practiced during the 1960s and 1970s, and the latter's proportion of use might have declined overtime.

The above pattern implies that in a society that is in the process of medicalisation, there is a possibility of home remedies and other indigenous systems of knowledge being overpowered by the dominant system. This, according to Panikkar (1992: 286), was also a feature of the colonial period when the allopathic system of medicine was first introduced in India. He argues that:

> ...the hospitals, dispensaries and colleges established by the state formed the nucleus from which colonial medicine sought to establish its hegemony and thus to marginalise and delegitimize the indigenous system.... [*the colonial state*] not only promoted western medicine but also sought to assert and establish its superiority over all other systems.

This is to say that during the colonial period, the state machinery like hospitals and dispensaries facilitated the hegemonisation of Western medicine over others despite the greater utilisation of indigenous medicine, resulting in the dismissal of the latter.

In a study by Saradama et al. (2000) on the extent of self-medication, especially antibiotics in Kerala, it was found in 69.3 % of the households at least one person consumed a pharmaceutical product during the two-week recall period, of which antibiotics formed 11 % of those products. This rate would have significantly increased by now. The study also demonstrates the overuse of antibiotics and increased self-medication trends of Kerala society as compared to others. The results of the current study among fever patients reveal that intake of paracetamol tablets with or without prescription for fevers of all kinds is a common practice in Kerala society. This was made obvious in the finding that 97 % of those fever patients who self-medicated used paracetamol or its derivative as a remedy for their illness. This implies the extent of dependence on a system whose beneficiaries themselves assume the role of expert while dealing with problems. It is possible that these behaviours can be legitimised in the long run, as is obvious from a patient's justification that 'as fever is dangerous and need [sic] to be prevented by whatever means of which paracetamol is an ideal one and is the one usually prescribed even by a qualified doctor'. This knowledge among the public that paracetamol is the medicine of choice for fever appears to be rational, but this has to be seen as an indicator that reflects the extent of medicalisation prevalent in the society where the *expert knowledge* of biomedicine has become a *commonsensical lay knowledge*. This feature, though it appears to be a way of empowering patients as it removes the physician from the scene, represents on the other hand a greater dependence on the system of allopathy that furthers the process of medicalisation.

4.6.3 Time of Seeking Treatment

Further, the mean duration for seeking treatment by fever patients shows that more (40.4 %) fever patients sought treatment on the second day of onset of illness, while a quarter (25 %) opted for treatment by the third day, and around 12 % sought treatment on the first day (George 2007). The fact that a majority (77.4 %) of the patients sought treatment within the first three days of the onset of the illness indicates not only greater access and utilisation patterns of health services in the society but also greater health consciousness among the people and a prompt treatment-seeking behaviour pattern. This behaviour of seeking treatment in an allopathic hospital within the first three days of the onset of a minor illness like fever has to be seen as a move towards preventive health behaviours, which for a self-limiting illness becomes unnecessary whereas in an epidemic it constitutes preferred behaviour. Examined in the current context, this is also a response to the fear of fevers that prevails in the society, thus triggering treatment-seeking behaviour. This was also reasserted from the perception of fevers by patients during and after illness, wherein most of them feared that the illness they were suffering could be any epidemic but after the illness felt that it was a 'simple fever' that could be cured without any drugs. It is important to examine this fear factor towards illness, as it is on the rise in Kerala state and also across other societies.

4.6.4 Number of Hospitals Visited Per Episode

Another characteristic of Kerala society in terms of treatment-seeking behaviour is about the number of hospitals visited by patients for fever care. It was found that around 23 % of the total patients ($n = 151$) surveyed have consulted more than one hospital or general practitioner for a single episode of fever. When examined further it was found that the mean duration among them was less than two weeks. If duration can be taken as a proxy for severity, then it is important to note what could be the potential reasons for changing hospitals for a minor illness like fever. Deeper investigation revealed that most of the patients who shifted to a different facility were the ones who finally sought treatment and were cured from the private hospitals at the secondary level, and that the shifting was predominantly from a primary-level private hospital to a secondary-level private hospital. This indicates that there are people who have multiple options in terms of access to health care for whom greater quality is valued and sought after. This also implies that there are several primary-level private hospitals that cannot satisfy the 'quality' needs of patients by providing care even for minor illnesses like fever.

The other pattern of shifting was from the public to private and private to public hospital, predominantly among the poor. This is to say that the poor shifted between the public and private sector more frequently depending on the context. Despite public hospitals being open to all, they often fail to ensure economically cheaper services, as many of the services (i.e. laboratory services and drugs) are provided by the private sector, for which the patients had to pay. This situation can result in the poor patients seeking treatment from the private sector when the public sector fails to provide its threshold services. This feature was also found in other studies that examined the factors influencing treatment-seeking behaviour for illnesses (Rao et al. 2005). This possibility increases when we examine the hospital procedures comprising the nature of diagnosis, admission pattern, prescription pattern of laboratory tests, and finally, the medical expenditure at various hospitals with respect to their sector and the level to which it belongs.

4.6.5 Interpreting Illness Behaviour

The above section on illness behaviour of fever patients reveals how the subjective risk perception gets translated into a form of medicalisation, wherein the changing pattern of managing fevers using home remedies to that of self-medication is an indication of how a certain illness that was once managed at home without any specific medical assistance is now treated under the purview of medicine. Further, the common sense knowledge of consuming paracetamol as the drug of choice for a range of fevers is also an indication of how people in their day-to-day engagement translate expert knowledge and practices into their daily life choices. These behaviours indicate greater health orientation to and acceptance of biomedicine within the society. Moreover, the greater access and utilisation of health care facilities in the state is obvious from the shorter time duration for seeking treatment and use of more than one health facility by a significant proportion of people for a minor illness like fever. In short, on one hand there is a clear shift of people's behaviour that signifies that the society embraces 'modern' medicine over their traditional ways, and on the other hand too much dependence on 'modern medicine' also exists, resulting in over-medicalisation, 'doctor-shopping', and so on, even for minor illnesses like fevers.

4.7 Provisioning of Medical Care

In any society, provisioning of medical care is cardinal, as its nature reflects the prevalent socio-economic and political forces and is a strong determinant of access to medical care. Hence, provisioning has to be examined within the larger context of social, economic, and political structures and policies followed by any country over time (Navarro 1975). In the present section, provisioning will be examined in the context of the changing government policies and programmes of India, as the study was confined only to one of the states within. Provisioning of medical care will be dealt with at two levels, the public and private sector on one hand and the areas of primary, secondary, and tertiary care on the other. This is because medical care at different levels has to be in tune with the kind of health problems prevalent in the society and the feasibility to offer it at a universal level. It is argued that in India, the state played a central role in finance, provisioning, and administration of health services during the early periods of the nation's formation—a role whose intensity has declined over time (Baru 1998). This does not mean that the state was the sole provider of service; rather, private practitioners have always been a significant group in rendering primary care, which is true even today. The Bhore committee, the blue print for development of health services, recommended universal access to basic health services to each citizen irrespective of their ability to pay (Government of India 1946). The Bhore committee and the then-prevalent notion of the welfare state providing social services were a guiding force in the health planning of India during the 1950s and 1960s, though its final implementation failed to achieve the desired results (Banerji 1985). During the 1970s, the threat of communicable diseases and the shortage of trained practitioners were a problem at the domestic level, and alongside the global recession, resulted in the shift away from the development of comprehensive primary health care services. The investment in health was more on medical education, training, and the specific vertical programmes for disease control, and this has retarded the growth of public health services in the country (Banerji 1985). It is at this juncture that the shift in the policies already guided by the then-prevalent *trickle-down* theory of economic growth along with sections of the population demanding hi-tech hospitals set the stage for the growth of the private sector (Baru 1998; Qadeer 2000). The already weakened public sector along with the state-supported private health sector, pre-dominantly initiated by the voluntary sector, together influenced the state of medical care in the country dramatically. Additionally, the various committee reports that inadequately addressed the nature and characteristics of the private sector remained a green signal for the growth of private sector that was also true of the pharmaceutical and medical equipment industry (Baru 1998).

The introduction of health sector reforms during the 1990s acted as a greater burden for the already constrained public sector. The major consequences were cuts in public sector investment, donor-driven priorities, and privatisation of medical care (Qadeer 2000). This is because there was a shortage of funds for the devel-opment of infrastructure at the level of secondary and tertiary care, whereas at the primary level, investing in already deteriorated primary health centres was con-sidered as resource wastage. The changing global context that allowed entry of multinationals to the health industry at a greater pace also shifted the focus from primary-level care to secondary- and tertiary-level care, wherein non-communicable diseases (lifestyle diseases) were highlighted as the major problem (Qadeer 2000). Not only were secondary- and tertiary-level private care highlighted as the choice for non-communicable disease care, but they were also *perceived* by the middle class as the *ideal standard* of health care. Here, it is important to quote Renaud (1978: 569):

> The capitalist industrial growth both creates health needs and institutionalise … [whose] mechanism is the medical engineering model, which transforms health needs into com-modities for a specific economic market. When the state intervenes, it is bound to act so as to further commodify health needs, thus favouring the unparalleled expansion of a sector of the civilian economy to the profit of those who capitalises on it, and thus further alienating individuals from control over their bodies and mind but without a significant improvement in the available indicators of the health status of the population.

This implies that when the state itself becomes constrained by capitalist growth, the state-propagated medical care that uses its own machinery can also become an institution that further *medicalises* the society, thereby catalysing the dependence on medicine. This is despite the proven case of medicine's incapability to solve health problems in various societies (Dubos 1959). It is this approach that points to the need for a cultural interpretation of medical practice to understand how the *medical engineering* process actually functions in a specific context. Before that, a people-centric perspective to examine medical care is required, as planning and policies adopted by the government are aimed at the welfare of their citizens.

4.8 Fever Care as Provisioning

The study approaches fever care as a form of provisioning that examines the distribution of public and private sector institutions at the primary, secondary, and tertiary levels of care situated within the larger context of government policies in general and health care in particular. This is because government policies directly impact health services and therefore medical care, a major component of health services. Here, it has to be noted that the weakening of the public sector or the growth of the private sector has to be subjected to an analysis that incorporates government policies, the socio-economic and cultural context of the people who utilise these services, and lastly, the outcome of medical care. This is because the health service system was historically constrained by the vertical programmes devised for the control of communicable diseases. Subsequently, the impact of structural adjustment policies during 1990s along with the corporatisation of medical care, a new form of the medical-industrial complex, together have tremendously changed the nature and characteristics of medical care.

Several studies have examined the role of the state and the functioning of its machinery during an epidemic. Shah (1997) in his study on the 1994 plague in Surat, Gujarat, demonstrates how the strengths and weaknesses of the state are exposed during a crisis situation like an epidemic. He elaborates by arguing that the public health services were performing better to effectively monitor and render care that was accessible to the poor, the major victims of epidemics. This does not imply that the epidemic was well managed by the public health services. Rather, the study exposes the failure of the public health systems of that time to cope with the situation, as a bad reputation marked the functioning of the health facility as a whole along with other weaknesses of the state to provide adequate sanitary facilities, drinking water, and so on. Finally, the study argues that implications of neglect directed towards public health services tend to be precipitated during epidemics. The study examined biomedicine uncritically, attributing most of the problems that arose during the epidemic to the structural factors alone and giving a clean chit for biomedicine per se.

On the other hand, from a patient perspective, the factors affecting the access and utilisation of health services demonstrated the role of patients' socio-economic, political, and cultural characteristics. The burden of any illness can be seen both from the health services' point of view and from that of the patient and his/her family. Both become largely a reflection of the policies of the government and its provisioning, whereas in that case of the latter, the social groups to which the patient belongs have a tremendous influence on their access and utilisation of medical care. It should be noted that the notion of quality of medical care, depending largely on the outcome, is a relative concept. This is because it largely depends on the context of medical care provided, patient access to the system, and more importantly, the outcome in terms of cost, cure, as well as assurance of long-term health. In short, health-seeking behaviour comprised of illness behaviour and treatment-seeking behaviour, as dealt with in the earlier chapter, has to be examined within the socio-economic and cultural context of the patients for adequate understanding of their access and utilisation.

Prasad (2000) examined people's access to health services during an epidemic of leptospirosis in South Gujarat in which he argued that access to health care services need to be seen largely as an outcome of the people's respective social spaces. He further argues that the context of suffering, articulation of pain, and sickness causation during epidemics has to be seen as a representation of other illness situations, since past experience with other illnesses as well as health institutions can shape people's behaviour during an epidemic.

This explanation of people's health behaviour during illness as examined by Banerji and Anderson (1963) in their study on tuberculosis that revealed how *worry awareness* and *action* during illness become cardinal in people's health behaviour. Going further, the study also demonstrated that *consciousness* about illness and cure and *action-taking* during illness depend on the prevalent health institutions and the patients' experiences with them (1963: 666–667). This understanding about health behaviour remained a guiding principle for a 19-village study that put forth the concept of *health culture*. Banerji (1989) defines *health culture* as the complex interaction involving health behaviour of a community, access to prevalent health systems, and the cultural perception and meaning of a health problem. Understanding these complex interactions is in fact an attempt to understand the social, economic, political, and cultural factors that contribute to the production of disease and access to health services. The study must be credited not only for its initiative to coordinate an interdisciplinary team to explore the varied facets of an epidemic, but also for the pioneering effort that aided in the planning of a national disease control programme.

4.8.1 Nature of Provisioning of Fever Care: A Population Perspective

A brief description about the various types of allopathic care rendered in the state will help us understand the general provisioning of medical care in the state. The types of allopathic care in Kerala can be broadly divided into the public and the private sectors. Within the *public* sector, there are sub-centres, PHCs, and CHCs at the *primary* level, district and taluk hospitals at the *secondary* level, and medical colleges at the *tertiary* level.

In the *private sector*, there are general practitioners (GP) and small clinics whose beneficiaries are mostly from the middle and upper-middle class. In addition, there are small hospitals managed by a single physician and at times two, who will be the only key personnel, with basic laboratory facilities and bed capacities of 10–15. These facilities are highly utilised by people from all socio-economic sections, especially the lower socio-economic class due to reasons of proximity, familiarity, and time saving (less crowded and evening clinics). All of the above facilities together form the *primary* level within the private sector.

There are also *speciality hospitals* where all the major specialities are available with modern high-end technologies like computed tomography (CT) and magnetic resonance imaging (MRI) scanners, echocardiogram equipment, and more, with bed strength ranging from 300 to 750 and wards of varied ranges, along with 24-h casualty facilities; these are comparable to the district and taluk hospitals in the public sector, and constitute the *secondary* sector. In addition, big corporate hospitals as well as trust hospitals that provide major facilities comparable to those provided by the secondary sector but which are known for one or two specialities also come under the *tertiary* sector.

Medical colleges with multiple specialities and teaching facilities constitute the *tertiary* sector. Public as well as private medical colleges function in the state. In fact, the boundaries between the secondary and tertiary sectors within the private sector often overlap, and it is difficult to make a strict demarcation. It has to be noted that though fever clinics were established only in public hospitals, the pilot study carried out revealed that the newly established fever clinics were not functionally different from the pre-existing OPDs. This led to a situation in which the comparability of the OPDs of the public and private hospitals at both the primary and secondary level became feasible.

It is obvious that the majority of the acute illnesses are managed at the primary and secondary sectors. Here, it is worth mentioning that the CHCs and taluk hospitals in the public sector and general practitioner (GPs) at the private sector are the ones who are forced to prescribe tests to be carried out by the private outside laboratories. This facilitates a market that aids the growth of the private laboratories in the state, due to the inadequate functioning of the existing infrastructure at the public sector (Varatharajan et al. 2002), as well as the fact that for GPs, a laboratory is at times non-existent. The above health facilities together with the district hospitals and medical colleges provide ample market for the chemists. In the private sector, especially at the secondary level, the hospital as a single institution has the autonomy of the market for laboratory services and drugs through which the division of labour and therefore the profit in medical care is ensured within its institutional limits. The treatment-seeking behaviour along with the expenses incurred during fever across public and private hospitals will be focused on below from a comparative perspective.

4.8.2 Fever Care in Hospitals

The process involved in fever care from the perspective of provisioning will be elaborated here. The analysis is based on the nature of the diagnosis that happened and the extent of admissions and lab tests prescribed in various hospitals as well as the total medical expenditures incurred across facilities. The four hospitals and their characteristics become important in understanding the provisioning of fever care rendered by these hospitals. As mentioned earlier, the four hospitals for the study were the *community health centre* (CHC) rendering primary care and the *district hospital* rendering secondary care, both within the public sector. Within the private sector, there was one hospital, Immanuel, a 700-bed hospital rendering secondary care, and Sivani, a 15-bed hospital rendering primary care.

4.8.3 Extent of Laboratory Tests

Laboratory investigations have become an important aspect of medical care in the current practice of medicine. The purpose of prescribing laboratory tests usually is to aid and fasten disease diagnosis. Since their inception, laboratory investigations in particular and medical technology in general have been projected as more of an *objective* means to understand the abnormality of human physiology (Reiser 1978). Recently, studies by Lupton (1994) and Atkinson (1995) have cautioned against the greater dependence of medicine on laboratory technology, as the use of technology per se does not necessarily guarantee effective medical care and can at times be counter-productive. This understanding was used in examining the types and characteristics of laboratory tests carried out among fever patients.

It was found that 57 (37.75 %) of the total fever patients ($n = 151$) selected for the study were subjected to at least one type of laboratory investigation. Among those subjected to laboratory investigations, 40 (70.18 %) patients were from private hospitals and 17 (around 30 %) were from public hospitals. It is worth mentioning that out of those 17 patients seen at the public hospital, eight of them received testing from private laboratories due to lack of availability of lab facilities in the former. Thus, 48 out of 57 fever patients (84 %) who received laboratory investigations had them done by private facilities. It has to be noted that laboratory investigations for identification of the malaria parasite and Tubercle bacilli are the only investigations usually carried out in most of the public health facilities like the CHCs and PHCs, thanks to the national health programmes. Routine blood/urine tests,[4] which at times can be crucial for medical care, especially fever care, are not provided in most of the primary-level public health facilities. In the current nature of medical practice, routine blood/urine tests have become ubiquitous, and are provided by a range of private laboratories in the state even in the remotest areas. This has opened up possibilities for a nexus between the public hospital doctors and the proprietor of the laboratories leading to an unethical prescription of laboratory

---

[4]Based on discussion with the laboratory staff of private hospitals and medical college hospital laboratories, it was found that for any diseases with fever as the symptom, *routine blood and urine tests* comprised of the following are prescribed. In urine, albumin and bile pigment is looked for; in blood, the erythrocyte sedimentation rate (ESR), white blood cell (WBC) count [total and differential count (TLC, DLC)], platelet count, urea level, serum bilirubin, serum amylase, and *creatinine phosphokinase* (CPK) are measured. None of these indicate the direct presence or absence of any bacteria or virus, rather they are an indication of the physiological functioning of human organs (systems), viz. liver and kidney, and therefore these are also known as liver function and kidney function tests. These tests are carried out usually to aid the nature and type of treatment rendered.

tests. As the duration of illness and the kind of symptoms does not show a significant difference across patients who sought treatment at the public and private sector, one can infer that there is not much difference in the severity of illness among patients who sought treatment at the public and private sector. Yet, the proportion of patients who were prescribed laboratory tests in private hospitals was more than double that prescribed in public hospitals. This reaffirms the possibility of profit as an influential factor in prescribing laboratory investigations, a conclusion that becomes vividly clear when one examines the type of laboratory tests prescribed by the hospitals.

While examining the type of laboratory tests carried out for those patients, a majority (64.91 %) of them only received a 'routine blood/urine test'. Another 17.5 % had routine blood tests along with other tests. Leptospirosis or dengue and TB were each tested, respectively, in 5 % of patients. The dependence on routine blood/urine tests in contemporary fever care has become so crucial that any health facility without these basic tests is seen by the people as being devoid of 'basic facilities' for medical care. On examining the prescription pattern across hospitals, it was found that the private sector at the secondary level (Immanuel hospital) prescribed the highest number of tests as compared to that at the primary level (Sivani hospital). These two hospitals have their own laboratory facilities, which further raises the possibility of profit being involved in each prescription—a task that lies within the autonomy of the practicing physician—and is therefore a way by which the power of medicine is exerted and sustained. Further, it was found that around 96 % of those who were admitted (26 patients) underwent laboratory investigations, indicating the greater dependence on laboratory investigation in medical care. The purpose and relevance of these tests during fever care will be discussed in detail in the next chapter on the culture of fever care. 'Preventive diagnostics', the new marketing mantra for the corporate medical care industry is an indication of how risk perception in a medicalised society aided with technology can lead to what Armstrong (1995) indicated as the rise of surveillance medicine.

4.8.4   Total Medical Expenditure for One Episode of Fever

Medical expenditure is another important indicator that not only reveals the disease burden but also reveals the difference between the care delivered by the public and private sector. Moreover, a comparative analysis of the expenditure pattern between the public and private sector for fever care can be an illustration of the extent of commercialisation in fever care in particular and medical care in general. Here, medical expenditure is calculated as the sum total of expenses incurred during consultation, along with the cost of drugs, laboratory expenditure if applicable, inpatient expenditure in the case of admission, and lastly, the travel expenditure. This was examined across the four hospitals under study and compared. Table 4.3 shows the distribution of total medical expenditures for one episode of fever. The findings show that around 70 % of the total patients ($n = 151$) spent less than

Table 4.3 Total medical expenditure for fever care across hospitals

Total medical expenditure for fever (Rs.)	Sector of the hospital						Total
	Public			Private			
	Level of the hospital		Total	Level of the hospital		Total	
	Secondary	Primary		Secondary	Primary		
<100	20	21	41	5	8	13	54 (35.76)
101–500	11	8	19	8	26	34	53 (35.1)
501–1000	4	7	11	6	3	9	20 (13.25)
1001–2000	0	3	3	3	1	4	7 (4.64)
2001–5000	1	1	2	9	0	9	11 (7.28)
5000+	0	0	0	5	1	6	6 (3.97)
Total	36	40	76	36	39	75	151 (100)

Source Primary Survey, 2005
Note Parentheses denote column percentage

Rs. 500 during their illness, of which half (35 %) spent less than Rs. 100 for fever care. Most of those who spent less than Rs. 100 had sought treatment from the public hospitals, with an almost equal distribution across the primary and secondary level. Among those who spent between Rs. 100 and 500, most of them received treatment from the private sector at the primary level. Those who spent Rs. 500–1000 constituted around 13 % of the total sample, with more or less equal distribution across the public and private sector hospitals. The distribution was similar among those who spent Rs. 1000–2000, constituting 4.64 % of the total sample with almost equal distribution in the public and private sector. In the Rs. 2000 and above category, the cases are skewed towards the private hospitals at the secondary level, indicating patients belonging to greater expenditure groups, most of whom were also admitted to the hospitals as part of fever care.

The above pattern demonstrates that during acute illnesses, especially where there is no inpatient care required, the difference in the medical expenditure across sectors would be minimal. This could also be due to the fact that considerable quanta of services in public hospitals remain idle or non-functional, for which the patient seeking treatment even at the public health facility must pay. Scholars identify this as the *idle capacity of public hospitals*, a feature of public hospitals where the infrastructure facilities are not functional for a variety of reasons, esti- mated to account for around 30 % of these hospitals in Kerala (Varatharajan et al. 2002).

Two issues arise in the above pattern. Despite the minimal interventions ren- dered by the public health facilities there are populations belonging to lower socio-economic categories that utilise these services. The major reason for this is economic. Second, the private sector at the secondary level has become the high-priced-service category, earning more profits along with concealing the service of the primary level that has been doing an appreciable job, especially in rural areas. Moreover, the services offered at the primary level within the private sector need to be appreciated, as 86 % of the patients who sought treatment owed total expenditures of less than Rs. 500, of which 20 % belonged to the category of less than Rs. 100. This expenditure pattern also explains why a private health facility at times can be the choice for the poor in cases of minor illnesses. On one hand we have the public hospitals that fail to provide the basic services free of cost, and thus patients are forced to depend on the private sector for laboratory investigations and medicines. On the other hand, there are private hospitals at the primary level that provide comprehensive care for illness at an affordable cost along with factors like familiarity of the doctor and proximity to the facility that make them more attractive to the people. Moreover, the cost incurred at these hospitals when compared to those at public sector hospitals will only be marginally higher or sometimes even less depending on the nature of illness. In this context, it is possible to argue that even after considering economic condition as the primary criterion, there can be a *rational* choice for use of a private health facility by the poor. This raises the need to reconsider the categories of *public sector* and *private sector,* as there are wide variations in their functioning in reality as compared to the general notion that the public sector is free and the private sector is expensive. In this context, the nature and characteristics of illness and the access to health care facilities along with patients' past experiences together play an important role in choosing a health facility for treatment.

4.9 Heterogeneity in Private-Sector Health Care

Further, the heterogeneity within the private sector health care also needs to be understood in the context of commercialisation of medical care since the type of patients served, components of care rendered, and therefore the cost involved across private sector hospitals vary considerably across primary, secondary, and tertiary levels. The data on the duration of illness reveals that the secondary-level hospitals within the private sector cater more to those illnesses with longer duration as compared to those at the primary level. However, the components of care between two private hospitals were significantly different even among those patients with similar duration. Moreover, the final diagnosis reveals that the majority of those illnesses under study were minor acute illnesses that are self-limiting, which generally last for 7–14 days.

The second aspect is the nature of care rendered at the two settings, which reveals that secondary hospitals generally have more intensive interventions for similar kinds of illnesses as compared to primary hospitals. This was obvious from the greater proportion of laboratory investigations and admission rates among the former. The difference in the charges for similar laboratory investigations illustrates how background conditions affect the cost of medical care, leading to larger facilities charging more for an intervention than its smaller counterparts. This, along with the fact that empanelled hospitals can only provide cashless facilities for those with health insurance coverage, make the secondary-level, private hospitals a sought-after setting, where demand for admissions for those with health insurance coverage takes place more often. A detailed analysis of the heterogeneity in private-sector hospitals for fever care and its implications for the urban poor is discussed elsewhere (George 2014).

4.10 Commercialisation of Fever Care

Research into the provisioning of fever care reveals the burden that people face due to fevers. On one hand, public-sector health care is becoming less of an option for the poor, possibly due to the introduction of user fees and other expenses incurred at the public hospitals along with inconvenient access times and other quality concerns, whereas those at the primary-level private sector find it difficult to survive in the context of market pressures created due to accreditation and government regulations that favour the secondary and tertiary sectors. One of the consequences of this could be a tendency among the secondary- and tertiary-care private hospitals to treat minor illnesses like fevers with intensive secondary-level inputs, which is not always required. In other words, in a situation where the public sector fails to render services to its optimum capacity, there is a market for primary- and secondary-level private-sector hospitals in the state. There is a competition between these hospitals to provide 'quality' care that satisfies the patients. This competition is sustained by the primary-level health facility by providing services similar to that provided by the secondary-level hospitals, irrespective of need. Meanwhile, at the secondary-level hospitals there is a tendency to project its 'secondary-level' status usually through the type of investigations followed and greater admission rates while providing care for minor illness like fevers. In short, it is the wooing of the market through projecting high-end medical care as a 'standard' by the private-sector health care that results in a context for greater commercialisation and therefore higher costs in medical care. This is possible in the field of medical care, perhaps due to the unique nature of medicine, and needs to be examined in detail and understood through the culture of medical practice.

4.11 Risk, Medicalisation, and Provisioning

The multiple perceptions of fever indicate that it is perceived as a serious epidemic at the time of onset, and as a minor, self-limiting illness once a person is cured of the disease. This takes place in a context wherein there is a threat of epidemics with fever as a major symptom in a state with better access to health care services. The meanings attributed to fever by lay people reveal that their understanding is tuned both by their way of life as well as the messages put forth by the dominant biomedical understanding. This indicates the complexities involved in the notion of fever, where every understanding is rooted in its context and can be logical. These varied notions of fever can be seen as an interaction of multiple knowledge systems prevalent in the society and how each of them interact in the process and are at times in mutual conflict or in concordance, obvious from the commonalties and differences in the lay and biomedical interpretations.

The illness behaviour of patients reveals the extent of the dependence on and dominance of the allopathic system as reflected by the patients' knowledge about fevers as well as their self-medication practices. The clear shift of the society towards *medicalisation* is indicated by the replacement of home remedies by self-medication, the example here being the intake of paracetamol. This is also not merely a patient-oriented phenomenon reflected in the ever-increasing role of laboratory investigations in disease diagnosis. Admissions in hospitals are becoming a prerequisite for valid diagnosis, a hospital-specific characteristic that enhances the process of medicalisation and gets intensified by the introduction of insurance in health care, usually denoted by the term 'moral hazard'. The most disturbing part is that despite all these interventions carried out at the hospital, only 14 % of the total cases ($n = 151$) had a final valid diagnosis and 23 % resulted in the suspected diagnosis category. This implies that around 63 % of the patients were diagnosed only up to the symptom level. This is a feature of both public and private hospitals alike, where the usual explanation given by public hospitals is lack of time and lack of infrastructure facilities. The paradox is that even without a final disease diagnosis, patients get cured, which again raises the question of whether a final diagnosis is only the need of an epidemiologist and not that of the physician, an attitude shared even by one of the leading physicians of a medical college in Kerala.

The provisioning of fever care indicates that on one hand public-sector health services are still a relief for the poor, as reflected in their greater preference. In societies where access to health services is greater, the time (when) of seeking treatment appears to be more influenced by the nature of illness than by the socio-economic conditions. Meanwhile, the choice of health facility is determined primarily based on the economic considerations of the patients, the nature of their illnesses, and their past experiences with the specific illness and with the health facility that had diagnosed and treated them. The major reason for non-treatment of ailments during the early stages of fever was the non-seriousness of the illness, as also shown by other studies on acute illnesses in general (Dilip 2005). The medical expenditures incurred by patients and their comparison across public and private sectors and between the primary and secondary levels of the private sector indicate the extent of commercialisation that is taking place even for a minor illness like fevers. This could be an outcome of raising the existing 'standard' of medical care even for minor illness by providers that are competing in the 'market' for health care. Raising the 'standard' is generally done by offering a greater number of 'advanced' medical procedures while rendering medical care. These procedures are not always scrutinised for their relevance from a medical care perspective, even to say whether it is commercially driven. This is a unique situation within medical practice, as the onus of this question ultimately lies with the medical fraternity wherein the physician and the nature of medical practice are the authority.

This case study shows how a society grappling with the fear of an illness—in this case, fevers—emerged from the 'perceived' risk of death and as a result transformed into a medicalised society. In this context, raising the 'standard' of medical care by offering quality services is projected by the private health care facility as an inarguable need of the hour. In other words, a risk-driven medicalised society aspires for more and more health check-ups and medical care, which raises the 'standard' for medical care, and thus the society's needs are 'satisfied' by the dominant private sector health care through their provisioning. This is a reciprocal process, as higher standards lead to further medicalisation and rising aspirations of people for medical care. How medicine facilitates this process of medicalisation through its practice will be the subject of the next chapter.

References

Alonzo, A. A. (1984). An illness behaviour paradigm: A conceptual exploration of a situational adaptation perspective. *Social Science and Medicine, 19*(5), 499–510.

Aravindan, K. P. (2006). *Kerala padanam, keralam engane Jeevikkunnu? Keralalm engane chinthikkunnu?(Malayalam): A study on Kerala, How Kerala lives? How Kerala thinks?.* Kozhikode, Kerala: Kerala Sastra Sahitya Parishad.

Armstrong, D. (1995). The rise of surveillance medicine. *Sociology of Health & Illness, 17*(3), 393–404.

Atkinson, Paul. (1995). *Medical talk and medical work: The liturgy of the clinic.* London: Sage Publications.

Banerji, D. (1985). *Health and family planning services in India, an epidemiological, socio-cultural and political analysis and a perspective.* New Delhi: Lok Paksh.

Banerji, D. (1989 July). Rural social transformation and changing health behaviour. *Economic and Political Weekly, 1,* 1474–1480.

Banerji, D., & Anderson, S. (1963). A sociological study of the awareness of symptoms suggestive of pulmonary tuberculosis. *Bulletin of the World Health Organisation, 29*(5), 665–683.

Baru, R. (1998). *Private health care in India: Social characteristics and trends.* New Delhi: Sage.

Dilip, T. R. (2005). Extent of inequity in access to health care Services in India. In Leena V. Gangoli, Ravi Duggal, & Abhay Shukla (Eds.), *Review of health care in India.* Mumbai, India: CEHAT.

Dubos, R. (1959). *Mirage of health.* Perennial Library, London: Harper and Row Publishers Ltd.

Ekbal, B. (2000). *People's campaign for decentralised planning and the health sector in Kerala.* Issue paper presented in People's Health Assembly 2000 held in Mexico (pp. 1–7).

Fox, N. J. (1999). Post modern reflections on risk, hazards and life choices. In D. Lupton (ed.), *Risk and socio-cultural theory: New directions and perspectives* (pp. 12–33). Cambridge: Cambridge University Press, UK.

George, M. (2007). *Interpreting fever talk and fever care in Kerala's socio-cultural context.* Unpublished Ph.D. thesis, Centre of Social Medicine and Community Health, School of Social Sciences, Jawaharlal Nehru University, New Delhi.

George, M. (2014). Heterogeneity in private sector health care and its implications on urban poor. *Journal of Health Management, 16*(1), 79–92.

Ghosh, I., & Coutinho, Lester. (2000). An ethnography of cholera in Calcutta. *Economic and Political Weekly, 35*(8&9), 684–696.

Government of India. (1946). *Health survey and development committee (Bhore Committee) report* (Vol. I). Delhi: Manager of Publications.

Kannan, K. P., Thankappan, K. R., Ramankutty, V., & Aravindan, K. P. (1991). *Health and development in rural Kerala*. Thiruvananthapuram, Kerala: Kerala Sastra Sahithya Parishad.

Kunjhikannan, T. P., & Aravindan, K. P. (2000). *Changes in health transition in Kerala, 1987–1997*. Thiruvananthapuram: Kerala Research Programme on Local Level Development, Centre for Development Studies.

Loustaunau, M. O., & Sobo, E. J. (1997). *The cultural context of health, illness, and medicine* (pp. 145–162). Westport, CT: Bergin & Garvey.

Lupton, D. (1993). Risk as moral danger: The social and political functions of risk discourse in public health. *International Journal of Health Services, 23*(3), 425–435.

Lupton, D. (1994). *Medicine as culture: Illness, disease and the body in the Western societies*. London: Sage.

Mechanic, D. (1969). Illness and cure. In J. Kosa, et al. (Eds.), *Poverty and health—A sociological analysis*. London: Harvard University.

Mechanic, D. (1993). Social research in health and the American sociopolitical context: The changing fortunes of medical sociology. *Social Science and Medicine, 36*(2), 95–102.

Navarro, V. (1975). The political economy of medical care, an explanation of the compositions, nature and functions of the present health sector of the United States. *International Journal of Health Services, 5*(1), 65–94.

NSSO. (1998). *Morbidity and treatment of ailments*. Report no. 441. NSS fifty-second round, July 1995–June 1996. New Delhi: National Sample Survey Organization, Department of Statistics, Government of India.

NSSO. (2014). *Key indicators of social consumption in India: Health* (NSSO 71st Round, January–June 2014; 2015: A8).

Osella, F., & Osella, C. (1996). Articulation of physical and social bodies in Kerala. *Contributions to Indian Sociology, 30*(1), 37–68.

Panikkar, K. N. (1992). Indigenous medicine and cultural hegemony: A study of the revitalisation movement in Keralam. *Studies in History, 8*(2), 283–308.

Prasad, P. (2000 October, 7). Health care access and marginalized social spaces, leptospirosis in South Gujarat. *Economic and Political Weekly*, 3688–3694.

Prasad, P. (2005 May–August, 2). Narratives of sickness and suffering: A study of malaria in South Gujarat. *Sociological Bulletin, 54*, 218–237.

Qadeer, I. (2000). Health care systems in transition III India part I. The Indian experience. *Journal of Public Health Medicine, 22*(1), 25–32.

Ramachandran, C. K. (2000). *Vydhyasamskaram (Malayalam): Medical culture*. Calicut, Kerala: Mathrubhumi Printing and Publishing Company Ltd.

Rao, S., Nundy, M., & Singh, A. (2005). Delivery of health services in the private sector. In *Financing and delivery of health care services in India*, National Commission on Macroeconomic Commission and Health, background paper (pp. 89–104).

Reiser, J. S. (1978). *Medicine and the reign of technology*. Cambridge, UK: Cambridge University Press.

Renaud, M. (1978) On the structural constraints to state intervention in Health. In J. Ehrenreich (Ed.), *The cultural crisis of modern medicine*. New York and London: Monthly Review Press.

Rothstein, G. William. (2003). *Public health and the risk factor: A history of an uneven medical revolution*. USA: University of Rochester Press.

Sagar, A. D. (1994). Health and the social environment. *Environmental Impact Assessment Review, 14*, 359–375.

Saradama, R. D., Higginbotham, N., & Nitcher, M. (2000). Social factors influencing the acquisition of antibiotic use in Kerala State, South India. *Social Science and Medicine, 50*(6), 891–903.

Sen, A. (2002). Health perception versus observation: Self reported morbidities have severe limitations and can be extremely misleading. *BMJ, 324*, 360–361.

Shah, G. (1997). *Public health and urban development: The plague in Surat*. New Delhi: Sage Publications.

Steele, J. L., & McBroom, W. H. (1972). Conceptual and empirical dimensions of health behaviour. *Journal of Health and Social Behaviour, 13*, 382–393.

Suchman, E. A. (1963). *Sociology and the field of public health*. New York: Russell Sage Foundation.

Sushama, P.N. (1990). Social context of health behavior in Kerala. In J. Caldwell, S. Findley, P. Caldwell et al. (Eds.), *What we know about health transition: The cultural, social and behavioral determinants of health* (Vol. II). Canberra Australia: Australia National University Printing Service for the Health Transition Centre.

Thankappan, K. R. (2001). Some health implications of globalization in Kerala, India. *Bulletin of the World Health Organization, 79*(9), 892.

Trostle, J. A. (2005). *Epidemiology and culture*. New York: Cambridge University Press.

Varatharajan, D., Sadanandan, R., Thankappan, R., et al. (2002). *Idle capacity in resource strapped government hospitals in Kerala, size, distribution and determining factors*. Thiruvananthapuram, Kerala: Achuta Menon Centre for Health Science Studies, Sri Chitra Tirunal Institute of Medical Sciences and Technology.

Ward, H., Mertens, T., & Thomas, C. (1997). Health-seeking behaviour and the control of sexually transmitted disease. *Health Policy and Planning, 12*(1), 19–28.

Weiss, M. (2001). Cultural epidemiology: An introduction and overview. *Anthropology and Medicine, 8*(1), 1–29.

Chapter 5
Biomedicine Examined: Interpreting the Culture of Fever Care

Abstract This chapter focuses on the culture of fever care within the context of medical care, in which the processes of diagnosis, prognosis, and therapeutics will be central. This is accomplished based on an ethnography of fever care within the microcosm of a hospital that comprises both administrative and medical functions demonstrating *medical work*. The process of diagnosis reveals how it is mediated internally by various artefacts like the medical record, thermometer, and the dominant role of laboratory investigations. This occurs despite the fact that a final valid diagnosis seldom happens in the case of fever. The claim of biomedicine that treatment is for the disease (causative agent) no longer becomes valid, as demonstrated by the cases on treatment modalities. These real-life situations where treatment is rendered even in the absence of any valid diagnosis, and antibiotics are prescribed for viral fever, all point towards the irrational use of drugs, an outcome of the irrational practice of medicine. Medicine has become more of an applied science, consisting of a pragmatically-derived range of disciplines and techniques distinguished by its specific purpose that ultimately separate the personhood of the patient from the medical discourse. This results in the classification of illness as a biochemical process or as an outcome of an organic lesion, where analysis and explanation are now the occupational task of the medical investigator instead of the earlier act of diagnosis and classification. In other words, due to its lack of scepticism towards the profession and its philosophy, biomedicine offers a cultural milieu for market forces to exploit the beneficiaries in the name of medicine.

Keywords Culture of fever care · Medical work · Ethnography of clinics · Medical cosmology · Diagnosis in biomedicine

5.1 Introduction

This chapter focusses on the culture of fever care, comprised of procedures carried out as part of medical practice upon those with complaints of *fever* (self-reported) to help the ill person get rid of the illness. The analysis will be carried out within the

© Springer Science+Business Media Singapore 2017   99
M. George, *Institutionalizing Illness Narratives*,
DOI 10.1007/978-981-10-1905-0_5

context of medical care in which the processes of diagnosis, prognosis, and thera-peutics will be central. The administrative function that covers the organisational aspect of the hospital and that can have a bearing on medical care will also be covered. The contemporary practice of biomedicine is situated within the historical evolution of Western medicine with special reference to clinical practice. In social studies on health, medical care generally implies provisioning wherein the pattern of care is rendered in public and private sectors as well as at various levels of care (primary, secondary, and tertiary), as dealt with in the previous chapter. This aspect of provisioning is usually carried out using empirical analysis, cataloguing the effi-ciency based on the audit of births, deaths, and health (Good 1994; Atkinson 1995; Lupton 1994). Vishwanathan (1997: 108) identified these as the *external* analyses that focus on the political economy of medicine, sociology of hospitals, or on the medical profession and that usually uphold some criticisms and reject others on *scientific grounds*. This renders a taken-for-granted position for the process of defining disease and a rationale for therapeutics, and thereby leaves the production of medical knowledge untouched. This inadequacy is rectified by several ethnographic studies on *medical work* that focus on the production of medical categories within a clinic. The present chapter is on the ethnography of fever care within the microcosm of a hospital that comprises both administrative and medical function, in order to demonstrate the *medical work* that has direct bearing on the outcome of medical care.

5.2   Early History of Biomedicine

It is not untrue that the history of medicine is as old as mankind itself. It is not the purpose here to provide a chronology of events that have contributed to the current biomedical practice, but rather an attempt is made to examine the major shifts that have happened in the theories of medicine and therefore the changing nature of medical practice. The changing role of the physician, patient, and the advent of technology will be given due consideration in the light of major philosophical shifts that have influenced the practice of medicine. Despite beliefs on supernatural theory, treatment was based on the causal observation that certain herbs could relieve certain symptoms. According to historians of medicine, it was a common feature that treatment never depended entirely upon orthodox theory during the early period (Cartwright 1977). Here, the effectiveness of the treatment was attributed to the faith of the patient towards both the drug and the doctor.

Ancient Greek philosopher-physicians influenced not only Western medicine, but also the Western world more than any other nation during this period. In 639–544 BC, the first theory of natural causes was propounded, which proposed that all natural substances including the human body are compounded of earth, air, fire, and water whose balance constituted health, while disease was treated as its imbalance. This became the basis of Hippocrates' (450–370 BC) *theory of humours* in med-icine, which dissociated medicine from philosophy by transforming a distinct theory that also refuted any role of supernatural causes or magic remedies. This was based on an experimental method lending a *scientific* outlook to medicine. Hippocrates was more of a practising physician than a theorist, as the patient was more important for him, and hence he was acknowledged as the founder of bedside medicine. He combined humoral theory with practical knowledge about anatomy and disease that together formed a true humoral pathology. To him, 'somatic disease was an internal battle between morbid matter, a concrete cause, and the natural self-healing power of the body' (ibid. 5). Later, during the century after Hippocrates' death, his successors rigidly differentiated medicine between five subjects: *physiology* implying normal function; *aetiology* or the philosophy of causes; *symptomatology*, which broadly meant the appearance of disease; *hygiene* or the principles of health; and *therapeutics* or methods of treatment (ibid.). The latter was further subdivided into surgery, dietetics, and pharmacology.

After the Greeks, the medicine known was largely of the conquerors who established their empire, first from the Romans when the Christian faith dominated the medical knowledge, and later from Arab medicine when translation from Greek and Roman texts were more frequent. It was during the time of Roman medicine that the humoral theory was rejected and the theory of *pneuma*, a vital principle believed to have been carried by the nerves and considered as the basis of life, became established (ibid.). Later, Galen (129 BC to 216 AD), a Greek who settled in Rome and was known for his compilation of the works of Hippocrates, accepted both the early doctrines of *humors* and *pneuma*. Though he followed Hippocrates in the method of treatment, he diverged from the earlier approaches of using single herb entities and began using complex herbal mixtures. After Galen, Roman medicine reformulated doctrines of *pneuma* and *humors* in a manner that gave final authority to God, as the Romans believed that humoral balance and *pneuma* were the spirit of God breathed into inanimate clay. Hence, the role of the physician was to alleviate illness and not to cure, as cures were miraculous (ibid. 11).

The Arabs revived the humoral theory and applied it to their remedies using two medicaments: sugar and cardamom, which were believed to have humoral properties in varied degrees. Their major contribution was in practical pharmacopoeia through the *alchemists,* who extracted the spirit from the substance (ibid.). After the wane of the Muslim Empire, the Latin-speaking priestly and upper classes began to move into southern Spain and translated Arabic manuscripts into Latin with the firm hands of the Church again controlling the medical philosophy. The firm hold of church not only forbade dissection, but also considered medicine an educational discipline totally divorced from the bedside (ibid.). The upper hand of church could not be sustained for long, as there was revolt against the repression of the holy church partly due to the scandal of rival Popes, and partly due to the terrible living conditions that developed in the second half of the century. The invention of printing and voyages of discovery during the fifteenth century widened the publishing of medical manuscripts, resulting in greater access to the works of Hippocrates and Galen for a larger group.

The sixteenth century was known for the contributions of two great men in medicine: Andreas Vesalius and Paracelsus. The former, known for his contributions to anatomy, passionately followed Galen's teaching to such an extent that any variation from the teaching was treated as a result of the changes that occurred after the first century AD, the period of Galen. His interest in anatomy raised the status of surgery to a science, which for Galen was *only a means of treatment* (ibid. 16). Paracelsus is known for rejecting the teachings of Galen and propounding a new theory of disease that identifies five causes: cosmic agencies, pathological poisons, predisposition, psychic, and divine intervention (ibid.). He had faith in astrology and alchemy, which resulted in the introduction of a number of metallic salts into the pharmacopoeia. Regarding treatment, it was believed that '…experiment was more valid than tradition, that therapy must utilise the *arcanum*, the potent quality of drugs to be obtained through chemical processes' (Temkin 1964: 3). Later, the battle between Galenists and Paracelsists ended by the complete disappearance of the followers of the former and the reduction of the latter to a small minority by the beginning of the eighteenth century.

5.3 Lineage of Contemporary Biomedicine

Until the seventeenth century, medicine has followed more or less similar ways as that of the early period following Hippocratic and Galenic foundations. The development of medicine was in pace with other sciences during this period as the Enlightenment brought a new outlook to society as well as to other sciences. It is also true that several important discoveries in science were made during this period. The major philosophical lineage of contemporary biomedicine can be traced by examining the history of medicine during the seventeenth, eighteenth, and nineteenth centuries. This experimental approach was the culmination of *inductive reasoning* and a *thinking machine* that resulted in the legitimisation of Vesalius and Paracelsus' followers.[1] In the field of medicine, Harvey's discovery of the circulation of blood and the theory of respiration resulted in the establishment of basic elements of circulatory and respiratory physiology by 1670 (Cartwright 1977). During the same period, the Royal Society of London was established in 1662 for the improvement of natural science, and the major physicians at that time translated these theories into bedside medicine (ibid.).

The physician's approach regarding diagnosis during the seventeenth century is obvious from this passage:

> To determine the nature of illness, he *(the physician)* relied chiefly on three techniques: the patient's statement in words which described his symptoms; the physician's observation of signs of the illness, his patient's physical appearance and behaviour; and more rarely the physician's manual examination of the patient's body. (Reiser 1978: 1)

The major focus then was the patient's narrative, and only in modern times have patients and physicians learned to accept diagnosis by physically intruding into the body. The location of medical practice was the home either of the patient or the physician, and institutional care in places such as hospitals was only for the poor

---

[1]It was Francis Bacon's inductive reasoning and René Descartes' proposition of the human being as a thinking machine (mind/body dualism) that set the worldview at the Enlightenment.

and the destitute. The meaning of hospitals then was quite different from the current usage.[2] Therapeutics during this period were under conflict between the Galenists and the Paracelsians, not only in terms of the introduction of chemical drugs, but also on whether to treat specific illnesses as entities or to restore harmony to the patient's bodily functions by restoring humoral balance. This was reflected in the writings during that period: 'Doctors treated fevers, fluxes, and dropsies rather than particular diseases' (Reiser 1978: 8). Upholding the argument of Paracelsus, Thomas Sydenham, an English physician argued that disease could be categorised into species capable of creating disorders coincident with their respective essences. He also proposed the possibility of categorising various illnesses into a finite number of species, class, order, and genera, similar to plant species. His descriptions of illness phenomena were based on the patient's story and his own clinical observations (ibid.). Sydenham's classificatory schema was later carried forward by several physicians.

During the same period, the social legitimisation of autopsies happened as the Enlightenment offered a new explanation about death and experiments:

> With the coming of the Enlightenment, death, too was entitled to the clear light of reason, and became for the philosophical mind an object and source of knowledge. (Foucault 1975: 125)

Morgagni, based on the autopsies he performed, published a five-volume book in 1761 that compared the clinical course of illness among patients with the pathological lesions at autopsy (ibid.). Thus, through anatomy, a linkage between the characteristics of the lesion within and the symptoms produced was established that also side-lined the search for the ultimate physical causes of illness. This report also helped the physician to ensure protection as well as increase his/her reputation by subsequent demonstration to the patient's friends and relatives of the true nature of the malady from which the patient was suffering (Reiser 1978: 18). Carrying forward this anatomical search, Francois-Xavier Bichat, a French physician, instead of attributing the impairment of the entire organ to disease instead considered disease as a local injury to the *tissues,* which for him were the building blocks of organs. He also added that observation of symptoms in the living patients without studying their effects on the anatomy in the dead was a folly (Foucault 1975: 131; Reiser 1978: 19). This idea of intrusion into the body in search of diseases not only side-lined the search for final causes, but also made the *site of infection* primordial. Foucault (1975: 140) commented on this as well:

> For Bichat and his successors, the notion of seat is freed from the causal problematic (and in this respect they are the heirs of the clinicians); it is directed towards the future of the disease rather than its past; the seat is the point from which the pathological organisation radiates. Not the *final cause,* but the *original site.*

The physicians too, influenced by the new orientation, shifted their focus from patients' stories and their visual appearance to the *internal* aspects of the patients in

---

[2]During this period the hospital was a place that provided settlement for the poor and the destitute, located as an attachment to settlements or parishes where *care* instead of a *cure* was rendered.

search of anatomic changes, which Foucault (1975: 146) describes as the shift from *clinical experience* to *anatomo-clinical gaze*. Thus, physicians' introduction of manual techniques as well as their search for tools for clinical diagnosis altered the nature of medical practice. Reiser (1978: 19) describes this as:

> The practice of dissecting bodies to find physical evidence of disease began to transform some eighteenth century physicians from word-oriented, theory-bound scholastics to touch-oriented, observation-bound scientists.

Broussais, in his 1808 treatise, explains the site of disease to be more important than the visibility of the lesion, as the disease in its nature being local makes visibility of the lesion possible only in a secondary way. In other words, it is not merely the presence of a lesion that is important, but also its effects that can disrupt the normal functioning of the body (symptoms). On this, Foucault (1975: 189) elaborates:

> With Broussais, localisation demands an enveloping causal schema: the seat of the disease is merely the link point of the irritating cause, a point that is determined both by the irritability of the tissue and the irritating power of the agent. The local space of the disease is also a causal space.

The above makes clear that Broussais identified the effect of any disease at two levels, the affected function and the affected tissue of the organism. Symptomatology, a sign of bodily functioning, at this juncture rediscovered its role but a role based entirely on the local character of the pathological attack. In other words, symptoms became a *means* to identify the lesion or the physiological imbalance. The purpose of therapeutics was not only to eliminate cause (local site) but also the *effects* that do not always disappear even when the cause has ceased to operate. The above explanation that the organism and disease co-existed in the same space nullified the *being (species)* concept of disease. This, in a way, provided a better explanation of the fundamental relationship between physiology and pathology (Canguilhem 1991). During the same period, the transformation from the study of *materia medica* to the study of *pharmacology* occurred. The tasks of pharmacology were to study the active substances within the drugs as well as the changes brought about by these drugs on the organism (Temkin 1964).

It was Claude Bernard, who deeply influenced physicians during the mid-nineteenth century, who argued that the continuity of pathological phenomena and the corresponding physiological phenomena are more of a monotonous repetition than a theme (Canguilhem 1991). He considered *medicine as the sciences of diseases, physiology as the science of life*. This, he demonstrated through his lectures on diabetes:

> Common sense shows that if we are thoroughly acquainted with a physiological phenomenon, we should be in a position to account for all the disturbances to which it is susceptible in the pathological state: physiology and pathology are intermingled and are essentially one and the same thing. (Canguilhem 1991: 67)

This led to the understanding that there are times when health and disease constitute one and the same thing, with the only difference being in their degrees. Extending this argument is the idea of health as the normal functioning (physiology) of an organism and disease as its pathological states (abnormal). For Bernard, 'any exaggeration, disproportion, discordance of normal phenomena constitutes the diseased state' (ibid. 71).

Almost during the same period, Rudolf Virchow, professor of pathological anatomy in Berlin, proposed the cell theory that later became the basis of modern medicine. According to him, 'the body is a cell-state in which every cell is a citizen' (Cartwright 1977; Waitzkin 1981). Therefore, the disease process causes normal cells to become distorted or to proliferate at an abnormal speed (Cartwright 1977). Thus, a new conception emerged of the body as a mass of cells, each one endowed with individual life and capable of undergoing change. This resulted in the understanding that as disease processes depend on the abnormal behaviour of cells, the cause of the disease could be found in the reason for why cells behave normally. It was Morgagni who identified disorder (abnormality) at the organ level, Bichat at the tissue level, and Virchow at the cell level. Even the contemporary search at the genetic level fails to explain the exact causes of several diseases. Yet, it was the cellular explanation of disease that led physicians to seek help from the laboratory pathologist in achieving their diagnoses (Reiser 1978; Cartwright 1977).

During the same period as that of Virchow, Louis Pasteur, a professor of Chemistry, identified through his experiment on fermentation a substance he called *germs*, which he explained as the cause of life and whose absence would leave all matter dead. At almost the same time, Darwin's theory of evolution was published in his work, *On the Origin of Species*. Both these theories questioned the age-old belief that God created Man, which resulted in one of the greatest controversies in the history of science (Cartwright 1977: 138–139). The discovery of germs by Pasteur led to the establishment of an association between germs and disease. Whether germs caused disease or germs were the manifestations of disease conditions was not clear until 1877, when he identified that anthrax bacillus caused death among animals exposed to anthrax. This led to the establishment of the theory that germs were the cause and not the product of disease (ibid.). Robert Koch, a year before Pasteur's experiment with anthrax, had already identified that anthrax bacilli can grow in animal blood as well as in tissues (ibid.). His continued experiments with microorganisms led to the famous *Koch's postulates* in 1882 based on his observation of tubercle bacillus. The *postulates* include the following: the organism must be present in the diseased body; it must be possible to cultivate the organism outside the body in pure cultures; and it must be capable of reproducing the original disease in susceptible animals (ibid. 141). The discovery of germs and the postulates of Koch were a new beginning in the field of medicine, not only in its *claim of scientificity*, but also to drastically change the very nature of diagnosis and treatment carried out by physicians.

5.3.1 Contemporary Biomedical Practice

Medicine that is practised today considers disease to be due to any abnormal variation in the structure or function of the body. Engel (1977: 130) describes 'disease as universal biological or psychophysiological entities, resulting from somatic lesions or dysfunctions'. In light of Koch's germ theory and Bernard's conception of disease as a pathological state of the body, contemporary biomedicine perceives the former as the cause and the latter as its effect. Thus the disease, in its manifestation, affects the structure and function of the body and can be identified based on the symptoms that render its signs, the knowledge of which is owed to Broussais, and can be treated with the appropriate drugs. Thus, according to Good (1994: 8), the tasks of clinical medicine are confined to:

> Diagnosis—the interpretation of the patient's symptoms by relating them to their functional and structural sources in the body and to underlying disease entities—and rational treatment aimed at intervention in the disease mechanisms.

Diseases are thus identified based on discrete sets of signs and symptoms or by diagnostic tests, which are categorised within the taxonomy of biomedicine primarily in terms of the biological characteristics of the causative agents. This ideal situation is more of a theoretical situation, whereas in practice the taxonomic and diagnostic systems are based on certain cultural assumptions about causality and normality; this is obvious from the practice of medicine that varies according to local traditions (Brown et al. 1996). Thus, the notion of biomedicine as that which provides an objective knowledge of pathology, represented as a reflection of the natural order revealed through physical findings, laboratory results, and the visual products of contemporary imaging techniques, is in reality an outcome based on the practical reasoning and work of the physician with the participation of the patient. These changes in the nature of medical practice need to be understood from a historical perspective taking into account not only the changing organisational characteristics and emergence of technology over time, but more importantly, the medical knowledge that plays a cardinal role in guiding this practice. This has been dealt with by several scholars, the most prominent being Jewson, who (1976) argues that the sick man disappeared from medical cosmology during the period 1770 to 1870 in Western Europe in the process of medicine transforming itself from being *bedside medicine* to *hospital medicine* and later to *laboratory medicine*. Furthermore, he attributes the disappearance to the change in organisation of medical practice from home to the hospital, extending later to the laboratory, which also resulted in the declining role of the patient in the process of overall medical care. Jewson (1976) considers these shifts as the result of change in the organisation and, using his terminology, the changing *mode of production of medical knowledge*, which in turn is seen as an outcome of the changing medical cosmology, where the concepts of disease, cure, and therapeutics are themselves transformed. Later, Armstrong (1995) examined a similar shift during the early twentieth century when normality became important and risk discourse within a population became the concern among medical care providers leading to the envisioning of a normal community accomplished through constant surveillance.

5.4 Culture of Medical Practice

The culture of medical practice refers to those acts of diagnosis, prognosis, and therapeutics performed by a physician upon a patient with an illness in order to help the latter overcome the illness. As mentioned before, this process (care) is ideally expected to follow the philosophy and logic of medicine, and is also called 'medical care'. Yet the culture of medical practice has never had a uniform nature and characteristics, as the context and institutions of medical practice have changed over time as well as within societies. The hospital here is considered as a microcosm shaped by structures and networks, ideas and images, and values and beliefs of the society and culture that both surround and pervade it (Fox 1989). Its medical functions include diagnosis, prognosis, and therapeutics, the basic procedures of medical care depending on the specialisation and infrastructure available, which in turn depend on the type of institutions.

The *medical function* of the hospital is of greater concern, as it is through this process that a lay category of illness (subjective) is transformed into a medical category of disease (objective) based on the therapeutic decision that will be taken. Moreover, hospitals are analogous to scientific laboratories wherein the production of knowledge (medical) takes place. Similar to laboratory studies (Barnes 1974) where the procedures involved in a laboratory are examined for the influence of *external* and *internal* factors, the practice of medicine can also be understood as that involving a *scientific* activity carried out in a hospital (Casper and Berg 1995). The *external* focuses on the political economy of medicine and the sociology of hospitals or the medical profession (Vishwanathan 1997). The *internal* examines the actors, artefacts, and procedures involved in the act of clinical interaction through which disease diagnosis and therapeutic decision-making happen. It is imperative to note that external and internal factors are closely linked. Ethnomethodology was used to examine them, as this provides a lens for closely examining the *everyday organised, ordinary activities,* of which medical care is one such social activity. Unlike other approaches, this does not assign a taken-for-granted position for any concept, be it disease or medicine's capability to diagnose and cure. Instead, it offers room for a close examination of the procedures and processes involved in the practice of medicine that identifies the actors, artefacts, and contexts involved in every event and how each of these influences the outcome of medical care (Lupton 1994, Atkinson 1995, White 2002). The purpose is to understand how *medicine constructs its objects*, using Good's (1994: 65) terminology, and how this construction affects patient care. Atkinson (1995: 45) agrees with the idea of a *social construction of reality* but does not prefer to use the term '*construction*'. This is primarily because the term has a connotation that questions the very existence of natural reality, and secondarily because he wanted to consider the *objects* of medicine as 'real' and not simply and solely a mental product. Instead, he prefers the word 'production', and thereby emphasises the *social production of medical knowledge* accomplished through *medical work* (ibid.).

No analysis of this sort can ever be independent of the social milieu of the actors and the health institutions, despite the fact that allopathic medical practice follows biomedical philosophy. Through this framework, not only is the lay category of illness transformed into an expert category of disease, thereby exerting social control, but the disease categories also add to the corpus of medical knowledge that guides future medical work (practice). Thus the major focus here is on the procedures involved in rendering care within a health facility where the social production of disease, therapeutics, and cure occurs.

One such study by Atkinson (1995) was carried out in a haematology laboratory dealing with disorders of the blood system, which is significant in the current practice of *laboratory medicine*. Atkinson focuses on how medical decision-making happens in a clinic in which the *actors*, *duration*, and *setting* all become important. He further examines how a patient (case) is produced in a hospital setting and how doctors' opinions must be analysed in the midst of certainty and/or uncertainty in biomedicine. Finally, he argues that medical work is a *socially organised ordinary activity* where the patient's body as an object of medical scrutiny is divorced from the personhood that is perceived differently at different sites based on the thought style or theory-laden nature of the observer.

A study conducted along similar lines was that of Good (1994), an anthropologist at Harvard Medical School, who applied an anthropological perspective to medicine and everyday experience. He argued that the world of medicine is a distinctive world of experience, a world filled with objects that are not part of our everyday world. Thus, to learn medicine is to develop a knowledge of this distinctive life-world, which requires an entry into a distinctive reality system that offers specialised ways of *seeing*, *writing,* and *speaking,* thus rendering it in itself a symbolic form (ibid. 71). For Good, medical knowledge is a medium of experience, a mode of engagement with the world. It is a dialogical medium—of encounter, interpretation, conflict, and at times, transformation.

5.4.1   Culture of Fever Care

The culture of fever care, viewed as part of the culture of medical practice, takes into account the prevailing medical knowledge during different periods, as this has strong implications for patient care. The major components covered under the culture of medical practice in this study were the modalities of diagnosis, prognosis, and therapeutics for those patients coming to any health institution with fever (self-reported). In this case, the study largely confined itself to the hospital as a microcosm, situated as a representation of a unit of modern medical practice. Here, the sector to which the hospital belongs and other supporting infrastructures like laboratories and pharmacies, along with the physician, the patients, and their relatives, together form the actors involved in the whole process of fever care. It must be noted that each actor and his/her actions and 'talk' together are seen as everyday ordinary activities organised in a certain way to attain specific goals.

5.5 Medical Record: A Vehicle for Accomplishing Medical Work

A concise definition of a medical record or case record becomes difficult, as a series of medical care activities are carried out by maintaining a proper case record. Roughly speaking, one can say that it is the record of the act of *doctoring*, comprising mainly information on diagnosis and treatment accomplished with or without the participation of paramedics. The significance of the case record was more for the purpose of *medical research,* as the content in the case record is usually seen as the doctor's description of a patient's distress (disease) based on expert knowledge. From a sociologist's point of view, it is through the process of documenting that the patient's illness gets transformed into the doctor's category of disease. Studies that have looked at the practice of medicine as *medical work*, have also examined medical records as a form of representation of the real work that happened before (Berg 2004). In the current approach, the role of the medical record is seen as such that *medical work* gets accomplished through this disembodied artefact.

The role and importance of the medical record varies with the person who examines it and the context in which it is produced. Its structure, form, and nature depend on the type of hospital (primary or secondary) and the sector (public or private) to which it belongs. A brief description of its nature, function, and characteristics as observed in the allopathic hospitals of Kerala will be captured here. In any hospital, the case record starts its journey from the registration counter where the name of the patient and the person's age is entered. Thereafter, this remains as the identification of the patient until he/she gets cured. In other words, it is this act that transforms a personal identity into that of a patient.

Once a patient starts consultation with the doctor, the patient's case record is kept ready in front of the table of the physician. Based on the description of the patient, the doctor checks the patient's name and age in the case sheet and then based on the format taught during medical training, the symptoms, history, habits, and so on will be recorded by the physician. Through this, the doctor prescribes laboratory investigations and other procedures if necessary. Then, in case of the patient needing laboratory tests, he/she has these done and returns to the doctor. By this time, the same medical record carries the *expert* message of the doctor to the laboratory technician, after which his comments are written sometimes on the same record or else attached to it in a specified format. Again, the patient comes back to the doctor and, ideally based on the laboratory tests, the doctor will write a diagnosis if one is found and then prescribe medications. In case the patient needs to be subjected to more examinations, especially from different specialities, all the details of their visit are recorded in the case record. Later, the same medical record reaches the pharmacy counter where the patient collects medicines and the pharmacist gives directions regarding timings for drug intake, the nature of the drugs, etc., based on the physician's prescription on the record. In the case of future follow-up, the same case record is used and the process is repeated.

The nature and characteristics of the case record depend on the sector to which the hospital belongs, whether the care rendered is of an outpatient or an inpatient type, and other factors like the type of doctor, type of illness, facilities available in the hospital, and so on. Despite these different factors, some commonalties and diversities were found across public and private sector hospitals both at the primary and secondary level. In the case of outpatients at the public hospitals, it becomes the responsibility of the patient to safeguard the case record as well as to carry it to various sites within the hospital premises and even to private laboratories and pharmacies situated outside the hospital premises if required. In the case of inpatients, it becomes the responsibility of nurses who are accountable to the physician in charge. On the contrary, in the private sector, case records are treated as *sacred*, and the hospital staff do not allow the patient or their relatives to go through (even to touch) them unless there is a strong demand from the patients and it is sanctioned by the doctor. It is interesting to note that separate staff members are allotted in most of the private hospitals whose major duty is to carry these case records to various sites within the hospital, and who are also the attendee to the physician. The *sacredness* or *untouchable* nature of the case records was further revealed during our fieldwork when it was found that one of the important reasons for which the doctor scolded the attendee was for allowing the patient to go through the case record. Similar to the case with outpatient records, for inpatients it was the nursing staff in charge of the patient who was responsible for not allowing the patient to go through the case record.

The above description shows how the case record accommodates various actors in its making. Further, this case record is treated as a valid document and the categories like diseases are treated as *scientific* categories in medical research. The division of labour among doctors and paramedics during medical care is coordinated through this record through communication among the *experts* without 'interpersonal' interaction. The *language* of communication is only understandable to those who are socialised to the medical world. The extent of work that the medical record symbolises becomes obvious when one considers that a single full-time staff member is employed in private hospitals exclusively to *transfer* the case record to various destinations as and when required. Above all, private hospitals do not even allow any patient to refer or to touch his/her own case record, thereby creating a barrier to its access. In other words, a sort of *sacredness* gets attached to the case record once the patient gets registered. This attitude is in its peak immediately before and after the patient meets the doctor. This *sacred* nature (possessiveness) reflects that once a person is registered as a patient in a private hospital, the autonomy of the hospital over various kinds of knowledge about the patient—for example, his/her disease, laboratory test results, type of drugs prescribed—lies with the hospital. The argument could be made that the hospital infrastructure made this knowledge possible and the patient *(subject)* is seen as a mere specimen (object). This autonomy over medical records is ultimately the autonomy over expert knowledge, which is reflected in its handling during *medical work*, as well as its procurement and handling at the medical records division, in the name of privacy and confidentiality of patients.

5.6 Diagnosis in Biomedicine

Diagnosis of disease is one of the major components of medical care, as it is through this process that a lay category (illness) is transformed into a medical category (disease). It is the diagnosis that determines the future course of therapeutics in patient care. Moreover, the *scientificity* of medicine is established by the systematic explanations of phenomena in terms of cause and effect, thereby formulating general laws where diagnosis is central. Samson (1999: 180) elaborates as follows:

> In medicine, laws appear in the correspondence between diagnostic taxonomies—names for ailments—and illness states, which are elaborated as to their onset, course, duration and outcome. Over time, through laboratory and clinical experience, facts accumulate and on this basis symptoms of disease, disease states and remedies can be named and entered into the knowledge base. The aim of these endeavours is to formulate predictive forms of knowledge so that facts about the body in general and individual clinical histories in particular can be deployed to predict the trajectories that illness will make.

From a biomedical perspective, diagnosis depends on three things: the *history* obtained from the patient, the *signs* noted on physical examination, and the results of *laboratory investigations* (Hampton et al. 1975; Wintrobe et al. 1974: 3–5). According to the medical literature, the ideal way of reaching a final diagnosis is the *syndromic approach* to disease where the clinical method is seen as an intellectual activity that proceeds from symptom to sign, to syndrome, to disease, in a linear progression from anatomical diagnosis to syndromic diagnosis and finally an ctiologic diagnosis (Wintrobe et al. 1974: 5–6). Data on the physiological and anatomical impairment is collected based on physical examination, thereafter tallied with the known facts of anatomy and physiology of the human body, and resulting in what is called the anatomic diagnosis. Subsequently, based on the above information and the prevalent signs and symptoms, a syndromic diagnosis is reached that does not necessarily identify the cause of the disease but narrows the possibilities that are capable of suggesting possible clinical and laboratory studies required (ibid.). Syndrome is defined as 'a group of symptoms and signs of disordered somatic function, related to one another by means of some anatomic, physiologic, or biochemical peculiarity of the organism' (ibid. 6). Further, it cautions by pointing to the possibility of the clinical method appearing as the scientific method, as it involves analysis and synthesis, the essential parts of Cartesian logic.

It is worth mentioning that it is impossible for the physician to start clinical work with an open mind, but only with one prejudiced from knowledge of recent cases, the patient's first statement, the physician's socialisation, and other factors that direct his thinking in certain channels (ibid; Fox 1989).

The role of laboratory investigations in the process of diagnosis is cardinal and so is the possibility of their influence in the process of medical care represented by the term *biomedicalisation* (Clarke et al. 2003). The prominence of laboratory tests and sophisticated medical technology within the whole process of contemporary *medical work* resulted in redefining diagnosis as more of a variation of numerical values than as a somatic distress. Scholars identify this as a characteristic feature of laboratory medicine (Jewson 1976; Atkinson 1995: 62), which Mccullough (1981) expands upon by examining the *thought style* that guides diagnosis and concepts of disease. He argues:

> that in a thought style that places increasing emphasis on the rational (and thus predictive) character of medical science—to put in an admittedly crude but accurate way, the contemporary culture of medical science—numbers and names take on powerful significance".

Thus, he further offers that laboratory findings often take on greater significance in determining a diagnosis than the findings based on history or physical examination. Once the physician has mastered the task of understanding the significance of these numbers, the physician is close to naming the disease, to make the diagnosis accurately (ibid.). Thus, medicine, with a highly rational and quantitative character, calls for a directed readiness for identifying the more *significant* result in a distinctive set of observations (Casper and Morrison 2010).

This could be due to the overdependence on technology in various walks of life —a feature of modern societies. In the field of medicine, this dependency is obvious from the tendency toward seeing numerical values as more *objective, scientific,* and *concrete*—first by physicians and thereafter by patients—becoming socialised into the same context. Vishwananthan (1997:105), in the context of examining the south Asian engagement with Western medicine, comments:

> …the laboratory test provides a series of readings…when seen as operational definitions of the reality of the patient, must have priority over the doctors personal impression of the patient as a person and the doctor's clinical impressions of the patient as a patient. The latter are parts of trans-science…sometimes dismissively termed as 'bedside manners'. The former allow for control and prediction and therefore [are] seen as the heart of the science of medicine.

The laboratory investigations in medical care not only act as an aid to diagnosis but also propagate the scientific nature embedded in medicine. The numerical values of laboratory tests can generate a notion of certainty among the physicians as well as the patients, which in due course can be transferred to the larger society as a whole. Scholars have recently identified that the perspective from the sociology of diagnosis helps in understanding it both as a process and a category (Jutel 2009).

5.6.1 Ethnography of Diagnosis

The real procedures of biomedical diagnosis are highly complex and are far from ideal in a textual description. A feature of modern societies is that many of the diagnoses in reality are confined only to clinical entities aided by laboratory tests and sophisticated medical technology. This feature gives prominence to the physiology of the human body, thereby neglecting the personhood of the patient. It is this aspect of diagnosis that makes it contextual and unique in its own ways, but at the same time subjected to the kind and nature of health institutions, prevalent knowledge about illness, physician's training, and more importantly, the nature of medicine itself. With this understanding about the process of diagnosis, two cases of fever that reached the health facilities are examined in detail with a special focus on the process of diagnosis taking place within the hospitals.

The first is a case of Kochumol, who sought treatment from a secondary-level hospital that has more than 300 beds, multiple specialities, and is registered under the charitable trusts act. The physician who examined Kochumol was a post-graduate in general medicine with 7–9 years of experience. The second case is of Shiny, who sought care in a small, 30-bed facility with basic laboratory support. The physician who examined Shiny was the sole doctor in that hospital, with only an MBBS degree but having been in the same hospital and practising medicine for at least 30 years. Ethnography of diagnosis was the focus here, treating it as a routine activity that happens in the clinics under study. Participant observation was used to capture the process of diagnosis during medical practice, supported by informal discussions with the physician, other support staff within the hospital, and with the patients and their relatives. Further, the medical record of the respective patient was also screened, which was an important source of data in understanding the meaning attached to the event by various actors.

The procedures for consultation in the hospitals is such that doctors and patients interact with each other and based on the patients' explanation, doctors record the details of the illness in a particular format in the case record. Subsequently, the patients are subjected to physical examination and laboratory investigations as the case demands, and thereafter are asked to meet with the doctor to discuss the results of the investigations. Then, the doctors prescribe medicines for a short period and ask the patient to come for a follow-up if required. The extent of physical examinations carried out, laboratory investigations prescribed, and other prescriptions depend on each case.

Kochumol, aged 29 years and a mother of two children aged seven and two years, sought treatment at Immanuel Hospital.[3] At the hospital she complained of

---

[3]Immanuel Hospital (a secondary hospital) has bed strength of more than 300, with emergency facilities and laboratory facilities capable of performing routine biochemical tests. There are specialisations for general medicine, paediatrics, ENT, ophthalmology, orthopaedic, skin and venereal diseases, and others. This hospital is especially known for its specialisation in the field of ophthalmology and cardiology.

fever, chills, vomiting, cough, and pain while urinating. She had a short consultation, as the physician found her very weak and then prescribed *routine blood and urine tests* before recommending that she be admitted. During follow-up later at Kochumol's home it was found that before going to Immanuel Hospital she had already visited a clinic near to her home from where an injection was given and she was sent back home. On the next evening, because of shivering and raised body temperature, she went to a physician near to her house, who also happened to be the physician of Immanuel Hospital. He gave her some medicine, but because she vomited the doctor asked her to come to the hospital the very next day, to which she complied. At the time of admission, the laboratory test results showed a low platelet count[4] (49,000/cu. mm). The report also shows the presence of albumin and pus cells in the urine. It was found that after one week the sickness subsided, and of the various laboratory tests only the platelet count was examined every day until the day (12th day) Kochumol was discharged from the hospital. The symptoms of the patient subsided after one week of admission and the platelet count was 100,000/mm^3 at this time, but the patient was discharged only after four more days when the platelet count reached 179,000/mm^3. At the time of patient's discharge from the hospital, the physician described the disease as, '*it was starting of dengue fever* and now she is okay'. During the first follow-up, which was ten days after discharge, laboratory investigations were prescribed and the patient's ESR[5] was found to be on the high side (120 mm/h). The physician then asked the patient to repeat taking the medicine he had prescribed earlier. In the subsequent follow-up after one month, a blood test was carried out again and the value of ESR was found to be normal.

The official diagnosis mentioned in the medical record was *suspected viral fever with reduced platelet count*. This was logical from the doctor's perspective, because medical intervention as a part of care hardly differs in the case of viral fever or dengue fever, as both are viral infections, and the approach followed is to treat the symptoms. Adding to this, the physician said that: 'the purpose of medical care is to relieve the sick from their illness and has minimal concern on the differentiation between disease categories, which is the job of epidemiologists'.

---

[4]This is because in most of the private hospitals, platelet count—one of the indicators of dengue fever—is used as the sole diagnostic test, which is strongly criticised. The normal platelet count per the medical literature can range from 150,000 to 400,000. Platelet count in the blood can be reduced in cases of dengue fever but this does not mean that all platelet count reduction can be due to dengue fever. Physicians admit that certain drugs can reduce platelet count, especially steroids, as can other conditions like specific cases of anaemia. For more details, see *The Hindu*, Oct 18, 2006.

[5]Erythrocyte sedimentation rate (ESR) is one of the *routine blood tests* prescribed by the physicians for patients coming with fever. The test implies the quantum of dead red blood corpuscles (RBC) that sediment in the blood. The normal value of ESR usually lies in the range of 20–40 mm/h. Though physicians consider a raised value of ESR in a patient as the presence of some form of infection, it is a general understanding among the medical fraternity not to act on a raised value of ESR alone unless indicated by other suggestive symptoms.

5.6.2   Medical Uncertainty Despite Laboratory Investigations

The above case demonstrates the significant role of laboratory tests in medical care, especially in the process of diagnosis. It was obvious from the medical record that platelet count was the only laboratory investigation that was carried out for each day of the patient's stay, and this fact together with the physician's statement that '*it is the starting of dengue fever*' demonstrates the dependence on platelet count in the process of this diagnosis. This took place despite the warning from the medical fraternity that platelet count alone cannot be used as an effective criterion for diagnosis of dengue fever, as platelet count can vary due to several different conditions and from the administration of some drugs for treatment.[6] The criteria for discharge also depended on the same platelet count, despite the fact that the patient's somatic sickness (clinical symptoms) had subsided much earlier. In the above case, the patient was discharged only when the count reached 179,000, the only value during the whole course of admission that was *normal* according to the medical literature. When the physician was interviewed, he said 'it is impossible for the practising physician to discharge a patient unless the platelet count becomes normal'.

A platelet count of 150,000–400,000 is treated as normal for humans according to the medical literature. Once the platelet count shows an abnormal value, it is associated with dengue fever, and blood transfusion is the medical intervention employed. Based on a discussion with physicians from public hospitals in the state, it was found that during the mid-1990s any patient whose platelet count was less than 100,000 was subjected to transfusion. Later, when it was found from clinical experience that patients survive even without transfusion at levels of 75,000, the criteria was lowered to 60,000, then to 40,000, and subsequently to 25,000. The dependence on laboratory investigations in the process of medical care, especially during diagnosis and treatment, is obvious here. This could be due to the physician's notion that more predictive power and *scientific* nature are embedded in laboratory investigations. Here, platelet count is the parameter that is depended upon judiciously by the physician. This test is not indicative of any particular disease; rather, it expresses more of the physiology of human beings. Furthermore, with regard to the ideal platelet count for blood transfusion, diverse opinions prevail within the medical fraternity. The threshold value considered for transfusion ranges from 10,000 to 100,000/cu mm. This again is a wide range and generates

---

[6]See 'Myths Prevail in Society about Dengue', *The Hindu*, October 18, 2006, p. 8. In the report Dr K.K. Aggarwal, president of the Heart Care Foundation, commented that though platelet count of more than 150,000 is considered normal for a person, transfusion is required only when the count is less than 10,000. He also warns that no painkiller or anti-fever medicines barring paracetamol should be given, as they can lower the platelet count. This leads to the possibility of platelet count reduction being a drug-induced abnormality, which alone is used as an indication for diagnosing dengue fever in several private hospitals of Kerala State, India.

possibilities for uncertainty during individual care. Here it is important to note that what is considered normal from medical knowledge can also vary based on contextual factors, reasserting the earlier argument that normality is situated in context. Thus, on one hand there is increased dependence on laboratory investigations that conform to the defining criteria of abnormality, whereas on the other, a proper diagnosis is lacking for simple illnesses that point to new realms of medical uncertainty within medical care. Fox (2000) identifies the various realms within which medical uncertainty is inherent and how this complicates and curtails the ability of physicians to prevent, diagnose, and treat disease, illness, and injury, thereby questioning the efficacy of physician practice. Here, the nature of diagnosis also changes in this context, as even in the absence of a final valid diagnosis (like dengue fever or viral fever), medicine is practiced in such a way that ambiguous disease entities like viral fever with elevated platelet count and ESR are projected in order to manage the uncertainty in diagnosis. It is through this process that laboratory results such as ESR and platelet count, many times a product of the interaction with emerging medical technologies, achieve greater significance within society.

5.6.3   *Vanishing Thermometers in Fever Clinics*

Biomedicine defines fever as a symptom characterised by an elevation in body temperature from the normal range, i.e. more than 99 °F or 37.2 °C (Petersdorf 1974).[7] Any description regarding the management of fever specifies the significance of temperature in the course of disease as well as the precautions[8] to be observed in using a thermometer. This is obvious from the textbook on internal medicine prescribed for medical students, which says, 'In fact, fever is such a sensitive and reliable indicator of the presence of disease that thermometry is probably the commonest clinical procedure in use' (ibid. 48).

Here is a case of Shiny, 32 years old, educated and a mother of twin children aged three years, who sought treatment at Sivani Hospital[9] for fever, headache, and

---

[7]Also, per the protocol brought out by the Directorate of Medical Education, Government of Kerala, in the context of fever epidemics, the term used was *syndrome of fever*, which attributed to fever characteristics that are more than a symptom. For details see, Government of Kerala (2004): *Draft Protocol for Syndrome of Fever*, Directorate of Medical Education, Kerala.

[8]A section in the document brought out during the epidemic gives a detailed description of the care taken while measuring temperature: the need to correct the mercury column, the time period for which the thermometer is to be placed inside the mouth, and so on. For more details see, Government of Kerala (2004): *Draft Protocol for Syndrome of Fever*, Directorate of Medical Education, Kerala.

[9]Sivani Hospital is functioning in a building that was earlier a house, now modified into a hospital, which itself gives a different outlook to the whole institution. The hospital is very old, run by a single doctor who started his practice during the 1970s with a good reputation of being simple and effective in medical care and who is popular for his humane approach.

cough. When she consulted the physician at the hospital for the first time she was suffering from fever, headache, cough, and body pain. The physician did a physical examination, used a stethoscope, measured her temperature, which was 102 °F, and prescribed medicines for three days. On her second visit to the hospital, which was after three days, the doctor inquired about her health and she reported having a severe headache and pain on the sides of her nose. The doctor again checked her temperature and found it to be 100 °F. The doctor then prescribed routine laboratory tests and medicines for three more days. On her third visit, Shiny said she was feeling better. The doctor on further examination found that her body temperature was back to normal (98.7 °F) and then checked the results of the laboratory investigations carried out earlier. According to the doctor, the ESR value was slightly high and referred the patient to a specialist.

Later, upon interviewing with Shiny at her home it was found that she consulted further in a speciality hospital where she was prescribed vitamin tablets and some tonic by the physician, who said that there was a 'shortage of blood'. The first doctor at Sivani Hospital explained the diagnosis as fever and headache with raised ESR, thereby failing to offer a final diagnosis of a particular disease. The greater importance given to ESR in the diagnosis despite Shiny having normal temperature and feeling better in the latter visit is significant. It shows how even in the case of simple illnesses, an abnormal value of laboratory tests is considered to be of great concern and dominates the process of diagnosis, irrespective of the somatic status of the patient.

The purpose of the above case is to demonstrate the role of ESR, a laboratory test that is gaining popularity in society in the context of fevers during recent times. The consulting physician was one of the few who still uses a thermometer for patients with fever, which is otherwise vanishing from most of the OPDs of hospitals. It was found during our fieldwork that most of the OPDs in public hospitals no longer use thermometers in clinical practice. The justification given was lack of time. This could be partly true, as 200–300 patients may be subjected to consultation by a single doctor in four hours (observed in one OPD session) in many of the public hospitals. Even a majority of the private hospitals during their everyday practice in OPDs no longer consider temperature as an important parameter for fevers. This is obvious from the fact that the physicians neither use thermometers nor rely on touch-sensation while consulting a patient with complaints of fever. In this case, it is not a matter of time, as a doctor spends on average more than five minutes with each patient as part of consultation. The explanations given by the physician is that temperature is no longer a dependable parameter, as different patients show different patterns and if antipyretics were taken before coming to the hospital these will distort the picture. The above explanations are valid to some extent, but the process of history taking can solve the problem of prior medication.

From the point of view of hospital authorities, to measure the temperature of patients, an additional duty would need to be assigned to the attendant, which overburdens the existing staff. Moreover, patients opined that since the same thermometer is used to record temperature for different patients, there is a feeling of stigma as well as fear of using them, as the patients *identify* a possibility of *microbes* being transmitted from one patient to another and that all patients in the hospital are *microbe carriers*. As patient satisfaction is the current motto of the private hospitals, the use of a thermometer is conveniently ignored by projecting the earlier-mentioned *scientific explanations* such as the unreliability of the technique. On the contrary, the raised ESR value considered as an abnormality by the physician is also becoming viewed as a significant abnormality among lay people. This was indicative from the behaviour of several patients who consulted doctors for the first time with their lab studies that showed abnormal ESR values. More astonishing is the fact that most of them had carried out tests from private laboratories without any doctor's prescription. Thermometers are vanishing widely from the outpatient departments of hospitals while physicians are resorting to using raised ESR values as an indicator for the presence of an infection. A brief description of the history of thermometers and the reliability of ESR as a test for minor illness is thus necessary.

5.6.4 Body Temperature Versus Erythrocyte Sedimentation Rate (ESR)

During the seventeenth century, when the thermometer was introduced in clinical practice for the first time there were several arguments against its utility for clinical practice, of which the strongest was a lack of time as well as its unreliability (Reiser 1978). Wunderlich, a young physician, countered these arguments in 1868 after publishing a treatise on the temperature in diseases that served as a guide to everyday practice. He outlined the fundamental components of thermometric observation, the art of using it, as well as a description of variations of temperature in 32 disorders (ibid.). Similar to any other medical technology whose values are expressed in numbers, the claim to *objectivity* was also projected. The very act of measuring was also considered a simple procedure that no longer needed the expertise of a physician, thereby shifting the task from the physician to the *helper* or *the attendee*, wherein the latter would have no pre-conceived notions about the illness and would thus be free from bias, resulting in a more *objective* value (ibid.). Thus, by the 1870s, Wunderlich's treatise had elevated thermometry to a highly regarded diagnostic technique. Despite several criticisms, the technique has been widely accepted as an exceptional method that can aid in disease diagnosis. This is followed even now in several hospitals, especially during fever cases. A passage from *Harrisons' Principles of Internal Medicine*, the text widely followed by clinicians in their clinical practice, illustrates further:

> The temperature is a simple, objective and accurate indicator of a physiologic state and is much less subject to external and psychogenic stimuli than the other vital signs, i.e., the pulse, respiratory rate and blood pressure. For these reasons, determination of the body temperature assists in estimating the severity of an illness, its course and duration, and the effect of therapy or even in deciding whether a person has an organic illness. (cited by Petersdorf 1974: 56)

ESR is the measure of the dead red blood corpuscles (RBCs) that have become sediment in the blood. The normal value of ESR usually lies in the range of 20–40 mm/h. According to physicians, an abnormal value of ESR implies the presence of infection, which is one of the explanations for an increase in ESR. Thus, there are several instances where rise in temperature, used as an indicator of infection, is substituted by ESR as a seemingly more *objective* unbiased value (number) that is irrespective of a patient's characteristics and that lies beyond the patient's domain. Even though raised body temperature as well as a rise in ESR both signify the presence of an infection, the shift from the act of monitoring temperature to tracking ESR does not necessarily offer any additional efficacy to the process of fever care. Here, it is interesting to find that in the authentic text of medicine, the relationship between fever and ESR is depicted as follows:

> …fever is not an indication of any particular type of disease; rather it should be considered a reaction to injury comparable to an elevated leukocyte count or a rapid erythrocyte sedimentation rate (ESR). (Petersdorf 1974: 56)

This cautions us that it is unfair to treat fever as a disease; rather, it can be viewed as similar to other bodily responses to exposure to external agents, reflected through elevated ESR or white blood cell (WBC) count. Instead, all three parameters (fever, ESR, and WBC) are analogous responses of the body to externalities. This shift from the use of thermometers for recording body temperature to relying on ESR in clinical work has to be seen as a characteristic of the changing nature of medicine, from *hospital medicine* to *laboratory medicine*. Here, the microscopic particles (specimen) replace the personhood of the patient, where it is the former who aids in the medical knowledge production. Thus, by shifting to ESR, the purview of medicine gets shifted from the physician in the hospital to the investigator in the laboratory—more specifically, to the numeric values produced in the lab. It is highly possible that the corpus of medical knowledge in the future might attribute an upper hand to the use of ESR over a thermometer in the case of fever diagnosis through backing by *scientific* explanations. Then, it has to be seen as a case of appropriating medical knowledge according to the changing nature of medicine, rather than the other way round as is generally expected. Further, presenting the illness through laboratory results not only masks the exact diagnosis (a disease category) that can be offered by medicine but also halts its search. Here, the purpose of diagnosis is redefined as that which offers *disease states*, a complex mix of symptoms, laboratory results, and sometimes a prognosis, during situations where diagnosis fails to offer a disease category. The term *disease states* according to Engelhardt, Jr. (1976) implies a combination of characteristics denoting the state of a patient, usually a product of medical diagnosis expressed as a combination of the symptoms of the patient, laboratory investigations, and psychosocial behaviour, valued against the social norms and thus attaining meaning and legitimacy to the social world. According to Rosenberg (2002) this transformation of disease states is a product of the changing nature of medicine by the development of pathological anatomy and supportive medical technology, a feature identified since the early twentieth century. The implication is that even trivial laboratory parameters that give an impression of the state of human physiology become powerful over the symptoms and legitimate concerns in their presentation, thus generating a more scientific outlook to disease entities and therefore to medicine. This according to Vishwanathan (1997) is a concern, when pushing the practice of medicine towards a more scientific enterprise can compromise the core purpose of medical practice— that is, pitting the aim of healing the sick against the production of medical knowledge.

5.7 Treatment Modalities

Another concern raised about diagnosis is about its purpose. The general notion is that if diagnosis is the identification of the problem, then treatment is the attempt to resolve it. It is quite obvious that a well-defined diagnosis can leave the problem half-solved. Not only is the search for diagnosis a form of active response, but it is widely recognised that naming a problem offers the sufferer and his or her family a degree of control through certainty that must itself be considered therapeutic (Samson 1999). The purpose of treatment is to alleviate the cause of the disease whether it is a virus, bacteria, parasite, or due to physiological, genetic, and internal chemical malformations (ibid.). It is important thus to examine how the medical literature perceives treatment modalities during *medical work* in general, and during fever care in particular. Therapeutics is situated as only one of the components of medical care in which primacy of the practice of medicine lies in medical care as a whole. This is explained as being due to two reasons: (i) in contexts where many of the drugs available are not beneficial, and (ii) the realisation of problems that can arise due to the tampering of the natural recuperative powers of the body (Wintrobe et al. 1974: 6–7). The text elaborates that ideal treatment should strive for complete restoration of the patient's physical and mental health. This in reality being unattainable can turn attention to those interventions that can postpone the progress of disease or that aid in tolerating distress (ibid.). It is possible that the extension of this philosophy led to the shift from cure to care; the latter is now the key term in medical practice. Extending this, it is *natural* for a biomedical physician to pre-scribe medicines for multiple symptoms when a final diagnosis is lacking (for whatever reasons) as well as when the *syndromic diagnosis* shows the features of a viral infection.[10] Additionally, a significant amount of drugs manufactured by pharmaceutical companies are meant for various syndromes like pain, fever,

---

[10]This is because there is no effective drug for majority of the viral diseases, as there are only very few chemicals that can attack viruses within the human body.

malaise, and nausea, even when none of these are disease categories. This can also activate (catalyse) the above tendency of treating the symptoms. This approach to treating symptoms rather than disease categories is known among physicians as *symptomatic treatment*,[11] which is a feature of medicine practised in the contemporary period. Going one step further in the context of overdependence on the laboratory, it is possible to find treatment that is modelled to address the abnormal values detected through laboratory tests rather than to address somatic distress or any specific disease.

5.7.1 Symptomatic Treatment

Raghavan, aged 49 years and working as a mason, sought treatment at one of the hospitals complaining of fever, cold, and cough that had persisted for two days. After the consultation, the physician prescribed medicines and sent him to get routine blood and urine tests done from the laboratory attached to the hospital. The tests showed no abnormality. The doctor wrote the diagnosis as 'fever, cold, and cough for two days'. The consultation between the doctor and patient was as follows:

D: How are you?
P: Doctor, I am having fever.
D: Do you have cold, sneezing, nasal block?
P: I am having all of it…
D: Is there phlegm?
P: Only that is there.
[The doctor examined breathing with a stethoscope, checked blood pressure and temperature (99 °F)]
D: Do you have any habits? [By this, he meant 'bad habits'.]
P: No. [P's wife interjected: 'He used to smoke cigarettes for everything'.]
D: You need to test blood and urine, medicine is written for now. Come after three days.

The patient returned after a week, when his illness was completely cured. The doctor examined him and remarked that his chest was clear.

The above case typifies the less serious cases of fever that are frequently treated at clinics. Instead of making a diagnosis, the physician simply notes a range of symptoms. The absence of a diagnosis challenges the logic of treatment—whether it is aimed at the causative agent or whether it is merely 'symptomatic', that is, treating certain symptoms on the assumption that once the symptom is controlled,

---

[11]Based on personal discussions with several practising physicians during fieldwork.

the illness will subside. Since medicines were prescribed at the same time as laboratory tests (rather than being prescribed after getting relevant information from the test results), it is not clear how the tests were meant to aid in the process of diagnosis. Such symptomatic treatment was quite common in the fever clinics.

In the case of Sheeja, a first-year nursing student, the patient consulted the physician of her teaching hospital (District Hospital) complaining of two days of fever, cough, cold, and body pain. At the out-patient department (OPD), the physician examined the patient, diagnosed her with viral fever and wrote '?Viral Fever', indicating a probable case, and prescribed amoxycillin, paracetamol tablets, and cloxacillin along with other drugs. Later during follow-up, it was found that her fever had been mild and subsided within a week. On detailed inquiry, she reported having already taken paracetamol and ampicillin tablets before consulting the physician.

This case illustrates a common practice where antibiotics are prescribed for suspected viral fever even though they are effective only against bacteria, and not viruses. As Dr Aggarwal, then chairman-elect of the Indian Medical Association, pointed out:

> It is important to remember that not all fevers are due to infections and not all infections are caused by bacteria. The majority of the infections seen in general are viral and antibiotics can neither treat viral infections nor prevent secondary bacterial infections among patients.[12]

Despite knowing the risk of bacterial resistance to antibiotics induced by over-prescription, many physicians still persist in giving the drugs. As the above case shows, patients also self-medicate with antibiotics even though legally these medications can only be prescribed by a qualified physician. The above cases show the gap between knowledge and practice that exists during treatment: whereas a final diagnosis should be a prerequisite for initiating treatment, it seems to be incidental or irrelevant in the fever clinic. In theory, only an accurate diagnosis can determine the prognosis and therapeutics for any illness. However, this is not the case in the actual practice of medical care in the fever clinic.

The medical literature regards therapeutics (prescribing drugs) as only one of the components of medical care because, in several contexts, many of the drugs available are not beneficial and problems can arise when they interfere with the natural recuperative powers of the body (Wintrobe et al. 1974: 6–7). Further, an ideal treatment should strive for complete restoration of the patient's physical and mental health. If that is not attainable, interventions should aim at delaying the progress of disease or helping the patient to tolerate distress (ibid.). It could be an extension of this philosophy that led to the shift from cure to care. Thus, it appears natural for a biomedical physician to prescribe medicines for symptoms when a final diagnosis is lacking as well as when the 'syndromic diagnosis' shows the

---

[12]*The Hindu*, July 17, 2006.

features of viral infection, which is generally not responsive to drugs. Additionally, many drugs manufactured by pharmaceutical companies are specifically meant for symptoms like pain, fever, or nausea, and not targeted at disease-causing agents. In this situation, 'symptomatic treatment' becomes the norm and probably provides some relief to patients.

5.7.2   Demonstrating Macro Influences Within the Microcosm of Medical Work

Until now, the nature and characteristics of core *medical work* are demonstrated based on the identification of the hospital as a microcosm where the influencing factors are mostly manifestations of the nature of biomedicine propagated and practised. These factors are embedded in the philosophy and cultural assumption of modern medicine, which Vishwanathan (1997) identifies as *internal* factors. There are other factors like organisational, changing policies of government as well as increasing corporatisation, which he calls the *external* factors. The next section demonstrates the interplay between the external factors and *medical work* occurring in the microcosm of a hospital. The cases below highlight some of them.

Mahesh Kumar, a 14-year-old boy, presented to the CHC with complaints of fever for four days. The boy was accompanied by one of the health assistants in that area who was also the boy's neighbour. As there was a case of dengue reported near the boy's neighbourhood, the health assistant suspected the same for the boy. The interaction between the doctor and the patient was as follows:

D: What is your illness?
P: Fever.
D: Fever means temperature or runny nose, for how long?
P: Four days.
D: Do you have cough, runny nose?

The health assistant, who is also a friend of the boy's mother said: I doubt whether he has dengue

D: Who had dengue fever?
The health assistant: In the neighbourhood.

The doctor then prescribed a test specifically for dengue and also prescribed medicines for three days to treat the fever. The patient returned to the health centre after three days with a body rash and redness in eyes. After examination, the doctor found that the test for dengue was negative but prescribed medicine for another six days.

In the medical record the diagnosis was written as '*?Dengue*', indicating it as a suspicious case of dengue based on the initial finding. Later, from a visit to the patient's household, it was found that the child had suffered from measles, confirmed from another nearby clinic, and had recovered within two weeks.

5.8   Societal Discourse of an Epidemic Interferes with Fever Care

During the two interactions with the doctor, the proper diagnosis was not made possibly due to the doctor's presumption that it could be dengue fever. Even in the absence of any valid diagnosis medicines were still prescribed, which questions the purpose of a diagnosis as well as the rationale of treatment. Moreover, in a society where there is a threat of epidemics like dengue, leptospirosis, or viral fevers, and with fever being the major symptom for these diseases, it is highly possible that the physician can overlook a simple diagnosis like measles. For a doctor in this context, the decision of diagnosis may be reached through intuition, which in turn is influenced by the societal discourse on diseases.

Jiju Sabu, 18 years old and a first-year nursing student in Bangalore, the only son of a widow mother who was working as a junior public health nurse (JPHN) near her hometown, came to Immanuel hospital for fever treatment. His mother had told Jiju to come directly to the hospital on his way from Bangalore back home, where both of them would meet at the hospital and consult the doctor thereafter. Things worked as planned and the boy reached the hospital for consultation after an overnight bus journey (12 h). The consultation with the physician is given below:

D: What is your illness?
P: Fever.
D: For how long?
P: Around one week (to which the mother of the patient added: 'Doctor, he is in Bangalore and there is measles and fever everywhere. There are rashes on his back and he is not taking food'.).
D: (*After examining the rash*) It is not measles, and the patient's record shows history of sinus (*after looking at his case record*).
D: Please cough (asked the patient to cough).
P: Uh!! Uh!! (Coughing)
D: Um, should be admitted. You will have to take various tests and if the results are normal, you can leave.

The doctor then prescribed an X-ray and routine lab tests, and advised for admission. The resulting lab values were normal. During the patient's stay in the hospital, an IV drip (glucose) was administered and usual inpatient care was rendered. On the fourth day, the patient was discharged. The diagnosis in the medical record was fever and sinusitis.

5.8.1   *Preventive Diagnostics for Surveillance: Expanding Functions of Hospitals*

Here, it has to be noted that the mother's behaviour correlates to that of a medicalised culture, partly due to her profession and partly because of her concern for her only son. This is reflected in her awareness about the communicability of measles and her knowledge of rashes as its symptom. Moreover, the mother's comment that her son had a body rash and was not taking food appears to be based on the patient's explanation to his mother about his living in a new place (hostel life), as the patient was away from his mother at least for a week. The purpose of admission to the hospital was for better diagnosis and to rule out the possibility of any 'epidemic fevers', rather than due to the severity of the illness. For the mother, an increased health consciousness led to an increased *perception factor* about her son's illness. This was reflected in her explanation of the illness to the physician as well as her decision to consult the physician immediately after a bus journey (overnight) of 12 h—after which any human being would likely be weak. This case raises some serious questions: What is the proper role of the physician in handling patients who are highly consumerist? What is the purpose of admitting a patient to a hospital? Is it the seriousness of the illness, or for the purpose of carrying out an effective diagnosis? Should medical care be based on patient demand, when patient satisfaction becomes the meaning of *quality* in a medical-industrial complex? How far can a hospital expand its reach and justify preventive diagnostics in a situation when the risk perception is higher?

Anwar, a 22-year-old youth working as a salesman in one of the leading wedding centres of the city, presented to Immanuel Hospital with complaints of fever, headache, and cough. The details of the consultation with the physician are given below:

D: What is the illness?
P: Fever, headache, and occasional cough.
D: For how long?
P: Two days.
D: What is your job?
P: Salesman in a wedding centre.
D: Do you have vomiting tendency?
P: No.

After examining the patient's body using a stethoscope, the doctor asked the patient to cough.

P: Uh! Uh! (coughing)
D: Will you blow your nose?
P: Sometimes.
D: Never blow your nose (saying 'nose' and 'blow' in English).
P: Eh!!!

D: I mean never blow your nose (in Malayalam). Get your X-ray and lab tests done. (The patient comes back with the X-ray and lab test results and consults with the doctor.)
D: Steam inhalation needs to be carried out using Vicks. Is admission required?
P: Yes.
D: There is no need for that. Oral drugs will be enough and if you need admission, I can do that.
P: Admission is required, Doctor.

The X-ray results as well as the laboratory test values were normal. During the patient's stay at the hospital, his temperature remained stable and the diagnosis per the medical record was fever, vertigo, upper respiratory tract infection (URTI), and allergic sinusitis. Here, except for URTI, all were symptoms, and the hospital treated the patient with injections and intravenous transfusions. However, the patient was discharged on the fourth day.

Peter Thomas, 20 years old and, working as a salesman in the same wedding centre mentioned above, presented to Immanuel Hospital with fever and cough. In the consulting room there was a senior physician (Sr. Dr) who consulted with patients, and a junior physician (Jr. Dr) who had recently joined the hospital to assist the senior physician. The interaction between the physicians and the patient is given below:

Sr. D: What is your illness?
P: Fever and cough.
Sr. D: For how long?
P: Two days.

The senior physician examined the mouth and nose of the patient and thereafter examined the patient's chest with a stethoscope. The junior physician was in charge of the case sheet writing and was entering the details of the patient based on the interaction. After examining the patient, the senior physician turned to the junior physician and started prescribing medicines loudly for the junior physician to write on the case sheet: 'cough syrup, expectorant, paracetamol'

P: (Interrupting): Doctor, I need to get admitted.
Sr. Dr to the Jr. Dr: 'Ah… then write for admission', again continuing, 'Cosome expectorant, paracetamol …'
P: Doctor, this is to get a claim.
D: You'll get money, isn't it?
P: Ah—it is a mediclaim clause.

The patient was admitted, although a lab test was not carried out and he was discharged on the second day. During his hospital stay, his recorded temperature was steady (98.3 °F) and usual inpatient interventions like intravenous infusion and injections were given. Per the medical record, the diagnosis was URTI, fever, and cough for two days.

5.8.2   Moral Hazard: Insurance Coverage as a Driver of Hospital Admission

The two cases above were of patients working as salesmen in one of the prominent wedding centres in the city. During follow-up, it was found that all the employees working in that shop had health insurance coverage for which they paid Rs. 202/- annually as a premium. The criteria for filing an insurance claim included at least 24-h hospitalisation in specific hospitals, and then hospital expenses up to Rs. 25,000/- would be paid by the insurance company. If medical care were not availed from those hospitals enlisted by the insurance company then the money would be reimbursed only later after providing the bills and supporting documents. Thus, in case of any illnesses among the staff of the wedding centre, their preference would typically be Immanuel Hospital mentioned above, one of the hospitals listed by the insurance company. Moreover, patients usually chose costlier wards, as the costs were paid by the insurance company.

The latter case demonstrates not only the influence of external factors like health insurance but also the socialisation of a junior physician in a hospital setup. It should also be noted that despite the fact that the temperature of the patient during his hospital stay was stable, it was officially written as *fever* in the medical record (*scientific recording*). Later during follow-up, the patient said that the illness was a minor one and he was cured by the second day. His preference to get admitted to the hospital was because he had no one to take care of him at his residence, as he was staying away from home, and the conditions of stay provided by the wedding centre are nominal and sick leave is an entitlement for the employees. The above case recalls the earlier question about the role of the hospital and hospital care in the context of insurance companies entering the health sector that are already part of a medico-industrial complex. In other words, is it possible to render health and medical care as consumer goods where patient (consumer) satisfaction can be made the criteria for good quality?

5.9   Fever Care as Sub-culture of Biomedicine

This chapter examines the culture of fever care as a sub-culture of medical care in the state of Kerala. The historical analysis reveals how Pasteur's germ theory and Koch's postulate became the basis for explaining the *cause* of a range of communicable diseases (namely, malaria, TB, cholera, measles, etc.), whereas the theories of pathology by Claude Bernard seem to explain its *effect*. In contemporary times, the search that was started by Bichat at the tissue level has advanced up to the genetic level without adequate knowledge of what causes this change in the body constitution (Cornad 2007). This becomes clearer when one finds that for communicable diseases a causative agent might be important, but for noncommunicable diseases where multiple factors contribute, Bernard's theory—that pathology is the quantitative variation of the physiology—appears to be the guiding principle. The latter seems to be true not only for non-communicable diseases, but also in cases when a causative agent could not be found, especially for a range of illnesses with fever as a symptom.

Practising physicians in everyday life do not necessarily investigate diseases at the cellular level, partly because this calls for better infrastructure and time consuming and expensive treatment, and more importantly, because of its minimal contribution towards treatment. Rather, laboratory parameters that only aid in measuring abnormality (pathology) of the body are widely used in rendering care, thereby halting the search for potential causative agents. This tendency led to the practice of using lab tests like ESR, platelet count, serum bilirubin, and so on as benchmarks by which healthy and diseased bodies get demarcated. Thus, disease definition has come to depend more on these values wherein the purpose of treatment ought to be to restore these abnormal values. Further, abnormal laboratory values, one of the indications of a disease, have gradually become the disease-defining criteria, as in the case of dengue fever, where platelet count—once an indicator of dengue fever—is now widely used in Kerala as a test for dengue. Similarly, abnormal blood pressure, which was once an indicator of heart-related disorders, has now become a disease condition in its own right, namely hypertension or hypotension. Dependence on medical technology in general, and laboratory tests in particular, cannot be due merely to the market-driven commercial influence of companies that are the ultimate beneficiaries; the changing nature of medical practice guided by prevalent medical knowledge also contributes significantly to this dependency. This can lead to a medicalised society as revealed by the tendency among the public to have lab tests done without a doctor's prescription and to approach hospitals without any *visible* somatic illness. It is this dependence on medical technology and the aspiration for *normality* that neglects the real clinical presentation (illness) that was once the starting point of being ill. Instead, the definition of an *ideal normal* body based on normal laboratory values became the basis to define the characteristics of a healthy body. The growth of preventive diagnostics in the realm of medical care must be understood in this context.

The processes of diagnosis demonstrate how the very act of diagnosis is mediated internally by various artefacts like the medical record, the thermometer, and the dominant role of laboratory investigations. This is despite the fact that a final valid diagnosis hardly happens in the case of fever and how, at times, the same illness is officially recorded in one way and then communicated differently to the patient. The claim of biomedicine that treatment is for the disease (causative agent) no longer becomes valid, as demonstrated by the cases on treatment modalities. This is obvious from the real-life situations in which treatment is rendered in the absence of any valid diagnosis and in the practice of prescribing antibiotics for viral fever, where both point toward the irrational use of drugs—an outcome of irrational practice of medicine. This, according to Jewson (1976), is the characteristic of laboratory medicine when two hostile career systems—researcher and medical practitioner—converge. Moreover, medicine ceased to be a subject defined by its explicit and exclusive contents, and instead became an applied science, consisting of a pragmatically-derived range of disciplines and techniques distinguished by its specific purpose that ultimately separate the personhood of the patient from the medical discourse. This results in the classification of illness as a biochemical process or as an outcome of an organic lesion, where analysis and explanation became the occupational tasks of the medical investigator instead of the earlier acts of diagnosis and classification.

On one hand, the changing nature of medicine has meant that medical knowledge and medical practice are now highly dependent on the medical technology and laboratories that play a key role in their existence. On the other hand, we have the commercial and corporate forces that are ready to utilise the gaps in medical practice that are inherent to the philosophy of medicine itself. In other words, **due to its lack of scepticism towards the profession and its philosophy biomedicine offers a cultural milieu for market forces to exploit beneficiaries in the name of medicine**. In short, instead of aiming for a rational prescription of laboratory tests and drugs, it is high time to aim for **a *rational practice of medicine*** rooted in the ethics of medical practice. This should address the prevalent medical knowledge, the philosophy of medicine, and its logic of practice rooted in the primary aim of medicine, which is to help patients get rid of their illness (un-wellness).

References

Armstrong, D. (1995). The rise of surveillance medicine. *Sociology of Health & Illness, 17*(3), 393–404.

Atkinson, P. (1995). *Medical talk and medical work: The liturgy of the clinic*. London: Sage Publications.

Barnes, B. (1974). *Scientific knowledge and sociological theory*. London: Routledge and Kegan Paul.

Berg, M. (2004). Practices of reading and writing: The constitutive role of the patient record in medical work. In A. Ella, M. A. Elston, & L. Prior (Eds.), *Medical work, medical knowledge and health care*. London, UK: Blackwell.

Brown, P. J., Inhorn, M. C., & Smith, D. J. (1996). Disease, ecology and human behaviour. In: C. F. Sargent & T. M. Johnson (Eds.), *Medical anthropology: Contemporary theory and method* (pp. 183–219). Connecticut, London: Praeger. (revised edition).

Canguilhem, G. (1991). *On the normal and the pathological*. New York: Zone Books.

Cartwright, F. F. (1977). *A social history of medicine*. London: Longman.

Casper, M., & Morrison, D. (2010). Medical sociology and technology: Critical engagements. *Journal of Health and Social Behaviour, 51*, S120–S132.

Casper, M., & Berg, M. (1995). Introduction: Constructivist perspectives on medical work: Medical practices and science and technology studies. *Science, Technology and Human Values, 20*(4), 395–407. (special issue).

Clarke, A. E., Shim, J. K., Mamo, L., Ruth, F., & Fishman, J. R. (2003). Biomedicalization: Technoscientific transformations of health, illness, and US biomedicine. In G. Albrecht, R. Fitzpatrick, & S. Schrimshaw (Eds.), *Handbook of social studies in health and medicine* (pp. 442–445). London: Sage.

Cornad, P. (2007). *The medicalization of society: On the transformation of human condition into treatable disorders*. Baltimore: Johns Hopkins University Press.

Engel, G. L. (1977). The need for a new medical model: A challenge for biomedicine. *Science, 196* (4286), 129–136.

Engelhardt, T, Jr. (1976). Ideology and etiology. *The Journal of Medicine and Philosophy, 1*(3), 256–268.

Foucault, M. (1975). *The birth of the clinic: Archaeology of medical perception*. New York and London: Vintage Books.

Fox, R. C. (1989). *The sociology of medicine, a participant observer's view*. Engelwood Cliffs, NJ: Prentice Hall.

Fox, R. C. (2000). Medical uncertainty revisited. In L. A. Gary, F. Ray, & S. C. Scrimshaw (Eds.), *Handbook of social studies in health and medicine*. London: Sage.

Good, B. J. (1994). *Medicine, rationality and experience, an anthropological experience*. Cambridge: Cambridge University Press.

Hampton, J. R., Harrison, M. J. G., Mitchell, J. R. A., Prichard, J. S., & Seymour, C. (1975). Relative contributions of history-taking, physical examination and Laboratory Investigation to diagnosis and management of medical outpatients. *British Medical Journal, 2*, 486–489.

Jewson, N. D. (1976). The disappearance of the sick man from medical cosmology 1770-1870. *Sociology, 10*, 225–244.

Jutel, A. (2009). Sociology of diagnosis: A preliminary review. *Sociology of Health & Illness, 31*(2), 278–299.

Lupton, D. (1994). *Medicine as culture: Illness, disease and the body in the western societies.*, London: Sage.

McCullough, L. (1981). Thought-styles, diagnosis, and concepts of disease: Commentary on Ludwick Fleck. *The Journal of Medicine and Philosophy, 6*, 257–261.

Petersdorf, R. G. (1974). Disturbances of heat regulation. In M. M. Wintrobe, G. W. Thorn, R. D Adams, E. Braunwald, K. J Isselbacher, & R. G. Petersdorf (Eds.), Harrison's principles of internal medicine (7th ed., pp. 48–62). New Delhi: Tata McGraw Hill.

Reiser, J. S. (1978). *Medicine and the reign of technology*. Cambridge, UK: Cambridge University Press.

Rosenberg, C. (2002). The tyranny of diagnosis, specific entities and individual experience. *The Millbank Quarterly, 80*(2), 237–260.

Samson, C. (1999). The physician and the patient. In C. Samson (Ed.), *Health studies, a critical and cross cultural reader*. London, UK: Blackwell Publishers.

Temkin, O. (1964). Historical aspects of drug therapy. In P. Talaly (Ed.), *Drugs in our society*. Baltimore: Johns Hopkins University.

Vishwanathan, S. (1997). *A carnival for science, essays on science, technology and development*. Calcutta, New Delhi: Oxford University Press.

Waitzkin, H. (1981). The social origins of illness—A neglected history *International Journal of Health Services, 11*, 77–103.

White, K. (2002). *An introduction to the sociology of health and illness*. London: Sage.

Wintrobe, M. M., Thorn, G. W., Adams, R. D., Braunwald, E., Isselbacher, K. J., & Petersdorf, R. G. (Eds.). (1974). *Harrison's principles of internal medicine* (7th ed.). New Delhi: Tata McGraw Hill.

Chapter 6
Voice of Illness and Voice of Medicine in Doctor–Patient Interaction

Abstract Medical care achieves its salience through the roles played by doctors and patients, and is accomplished through their interaction. This interaction transforms a lay category (*illness*) to a medical category (*disease*) by providing an expert and lay interpretation of an event, which in turn reveals the context and the reasons for these interpretations. The present chapter is an attempt to examine these interactions in the process of fever care in the allopathic hospitals of Kerala. Narrative analysis will be used, as it can simultaneously be a tool to situate the physician and patient in their sociocultural milieu as well as a means of communication whose further analysis can provide the meaning given by both the actors to a common event, illness. Moreover, on close examination, the conditions of narrative production help us to identify the role of 'institutions' in construction of the social context in which narrative is embedded. Within this framework the concept of *voice* will be used, wherein a voice of illness and a voice of medicine are identified. The **voice of illness** can be divided into a *lifeworld voice of illness* and a *medicalised voice of illness*. Further, the **voice of medicine** can be divided into a *voice of science* and a *voice of experience*. All of these voices are used for the analysis of doctor–patient interaction in fever care. Different voices distinguish contrasting orientations to the world and to the moral order, as each voice realises a particular relationship between the speaker and the world. This analysis in terms of voice not only situates the clinical interaction as a dynamic one where the power of the patient is acknowledged but also portrays doctor–patient interaction as an everyday activity of human beings. Thus, it is argued that clinical interaction is not merely a form of two-way communication intended for the exchange of information; rather, it is also the product of the networks in which both the actors function, which in turn are the outcome of the socialisation of doctors (*thought styles*) and patients' (*lifeworld*) about an event (illness) within their respective contexts.

Keywords Doctor-patient interaction · Narrative analysis · Voice of illness · Voice of medicine · Medicalisation · Thought styles

Portions of this chapter are also to be found in Sociological Bulletin, 2010, 59(2) 159–178.

6.1   Introduction

Medical care achieves its salience through the processes of diagnosis, treatment, and follow-up. These are usually accomplished by the active group effort of doctors, patients, and other paramedical staff within health institutions. The roles played by doctors and patients become pivotal in the process of medical care. The role played by the patient cannot be seen merely as a recipient of medical care but as a partner in the total effort to cure a disease, as it is the patient and/or his/her relatives who first identify the problem and seek treatment. This becomes a necessary condition for the recovery of illness through medical care. Apart from this, the whole process of medical care that transforms a lay category of *illness* into a medical category, viz. *disease,* is facilitated through these interactions. In other words, doctor–patient interaction can provide an expert and a lay interpretation of the same event, which in turn reveals the context and the reasons for these interpretations. The present chapter is an interpretation of doctor–patient interactions in the context of fever care and thereby explains these interactions as outcomes of the socialisation of the actors involved.

6.2   Understanding the Doctor–Patient Interaction

The interactions between doctors and patients become cardinal not only in the process of medical care but also within the institution of medicine. It is through this interaction that the basic procedures of medical care like diagnosis, prognosis, and therapeutics are accomplished. This interaction can be a part of the whole process of medical care where both the actors are influenced by the changing medical knowledge. Several approaches can be taken to examine the interaction between doctors and patients.

The concern towards the medical profession in early times was predominantly from a sociology-*in*-medicine perspective where patients were viewed as having a passive role and were expected to co-operate with the doctor in the process of medical care (Seal 1971). These studies mostly examined the gaps in patient knowledge and understanding about medicine with a view to rectify them by the process of socialising patients to medical values and beliefs. Parsons' (1951) sick role has been one of the dominant as well as influential approaches among sociologists, which resulted in the acceptance of the physician's expertise in tackling illness as the key for doctor–patient interaction. This not only problematises illness but also considers bureaucracy in the hospital as a feature manifested through doctor–patient interaction (Tuckett 1976; Mechanic 1976). In all these, patients were not given sufficient attention, as the major role attributed to them was to help the physician to the extent possible in the collection of information about illness for rendering better care. From a professional perspective, another stream of studies examined the temperament, behaviour, and attitude of doctors and patients and tried to link them with the class to which they belong, thereby demonstrating conflict between them (Friedson 1970, 2001; Advani 1980).

Taking into consideration the varied roles played by doctors and patients, four models were developed to understand the physician and patient relationship. They are the paternalistic, informative, interpretative, and deliberative models (Emanuel and Emanuel 1992). In all these approaches, the upper hand and expertise of the physician and the capability attributed to medicine is obvious. The rise of the consumerist perspective that considers medical care as a commodity and the right of the patient as that of a consumer further attempts to empower the patient; as a result, the patient is expected to assert his needs and make himself aware of the possible options. This does not go very far due to the patient's inability to enter into the realm of expertise of medical knowledge, which plays an important role in the process of medical care decision-making. For Waitzkin (1979), this is the outcome of a professional hegemony embedded in medicine that is a characteristic of any society whose intensity is greater in a capitalist society, and thus is capable of exerting social control that ultimately gets precipitated through the doctor–patient interaction.

The realisation of uncertainty within medicine (Fox 1957, 2000) has resulted in an approach that questions the acceptance of physician expertise in tackling illness. Here, diagnosis itself is seen as a practical approach that does not seek to achieve more than a prediction of appropriate therapy and a theoretical approach that seeks to refine diagnosis to the limits of the possible (Mccormick 1979). Further, the reasons that people consult doctors were not always for diagnosis and treatment of disease, but also for reassurance about the meaning of symptoms, assistance with the problems of living, certification of sickness, and also prevention of disease (ibid.). In this context it would be farcical to understand the doctor–patient interaction merely as a dyadic relationship. Instead, a contextual analysis that situates *doctors* as the representation of the prevalent medical fraternity and *patients*, depending on the social strata to which they belong, as reflections of the prevalent cultural practices reflected in the *type of health institutions*, needs to be captured (Atkinson 1995; Good and Good 2000).

This can be a means for analysing how larger social and cultural processes are made relevant to the experience of patients, suggesting that clinical conversations are a form of traffic not only among doctors and patients, but also among diverse local and global sites that produce biomedical knowledge, therapeutic technologies, and the scientific imaginary (Good and Good 2000). This is to say that consultation is the forum through which biomedical theory and scientific assumptions meet *lay expressions* of the experience of illness. In the encounter, the personal, social, and psychological contexts of sickness that are brought by the patient are translated by the physician into terms that are intelligible in biomedicine. An understanding of this encounter is accomplished here by analysing the doctor–patient interaction in its totality using *narrative analysis,* engaging with its basic assumptions and techniques as well as its appropriateness.

6.3 Narratives and the Social World

Narrative as an approach for social inquiry has to be examined in depth to understand its potential as well as its limitations. The narrative approach according to Moen (2006) is a frame of reference, a way of reflecting during the entire inquiry process, as a research method and a mode for representation as a frame of reference. In other words, narrative can be a mode of knowing as well as a mode of communication about reality by contextualising events and thereby attributing meaning (Czarniawska 2004). The importance of context in understanding events and the cardinal role of context in understanding human behaviour is explained well by Schutz (1973), cited in Czarniawska (2004: 4) as '… it is impossible to understand human conduct while ignoring its intentions, and it is impossible to understand human intentions while ignoring the settings in which they make sense'. Another aspect of narrative that is relevant in current discussion is narrative as a mode of communication. A narrative paradigm of communication assumes that there exists a different rationality, narrative rationality, which calls for a contextual prerequisite for dialogue. Here, a concept of dialogue is implied that is not always between individuals but also with the consciousness and the self and with the surroundings.

Thus, an understanding of the social world becomes richer when these interactions are captured through narratives. Narrative allows us to make better sense of the interactions, since the close linkage between narrative and experience as well as the power of articulation through narrative has been identified as a better representation of the social world. Scholars (Czarniawska 2004; Moen 2006) have noted that life events can be better described through stories, in narrative form, since they are merely a depiction of lived experiences. There has been tremendous development in terms of using narrative for social inquiry in diverse contexts. This includes those inquiries within formal settings like educational institutions (e.g. schools and universities), hospitals, and prisons, along with informal situations like streets and marketplaces and other sites of human interaction.

Doctor–patient interaction is one such naturally occurring ordinary activity that takes place within a social institution, a clinic. This is a process by which a patient approaches a doctor to seek help for a problem, in a context where there is societal legitimacy for this action. Here, the narrative of physicians can reveal meanings about a disease, its causes, and its treatment from within a medical paradigm. On the other hand, the patient may articulate the experience of illness and the burden it creates both at work and at home, along with other concerns. Through narratives, it is these two perspectives that can be analysed in a given setting. Here, the patient category of illness gets transformed into a medical category—disease—thus transforming the subjective experience of the patient into an objective category of medicine. Additionally, narratives can demonstrate the negotiations between the doctor and the patient and the power relations between them, and can be subjected to critical analysis both as a mode of communication and a mode of knowledge production, by unravelling the ways in which background factors condition the practice of medicine. It is in this context of viewing narrative as a mode of communication that the concept of voice attains greater significance.

6.4 Narrative Analysis of the Doctor–Patient Interaction

The suitability of narrative analysis in clinical encounters is dealt with by Mattingly (1994: 811) as follows: 'Narrative plays a central role in clinical work not only as a retrospective account of past events but as a form healers and patients actively seek to impose upon clinical time'. This becomes clear as (illness) narratives are extensively used to understand patients' representations and experiences of illness as well as to provide a temporal frame (clinical time) for therapeutic events. When the doctor–patient interaction is seen as a narrative, the scope of analysis widens, thus transforming the moment into a tool with which to situate the physician and patient in their sociocultural milieu. It also becomes a means of communication whose further analysis provides the meaning given by both the actors to a common event, viz., illness. This is because narrative can be studied as a mode of discourse —as text or as performance (Mattingly 1994). This is further clarified by Mattingly and Garro: 'Narrative is used when we want to understand concrete events that require relating an inner world of desire and motive to an outer world of observable actions and states of affairs' (1994: 771).

Narrative thus makes it possible to understand not only past experiences but through them the present understanding of that experience, as well as the future options perceived within the given sociocultural context. As *narrative* is about *experiences*, it is through stories that narratives are produced, where stories themselves are outcomes of experiences of the actors within their respective context (socialisation). The linkages between narrative and life stories have been dealt with extensively by many scholars, the details of which would be inappropriate to include at this juncture (Mattingly and Garro 2000; Frank 1995). It is this narrative or life stories that are further analysed by the researcher as a *text* based on the researcher's sociocultural milieu (socialisation). Thus, the model in which *experience* leads to *narrative* and narrative to *text* and text further reshapes the experience is in itself inadequate, as the role of socialisation of the actors as well as the researcher in the formation of narrative as well as the text is not adequately addressed. This inadequacy is tackled by introducing the concept of *institutions* at each juncture—that is, during the translation of *experience* to *narrative* and narrative to *text* and text further reshaping the experience. The concept of *institutions* used for this study is based on Saris' (1995) work about a schizophrenic patient whose details are laid out in the next section.

6.5 Situating Institutions in Illness Narratives

Saris (1995) in his paper on illness narratives addressed the above problem by elaborating narrative, or in his terminology, *the conditions of narrative production,* more convincingly. The translation of *experience* to *narrative* and narrative to *text* according to Saris is shaped by the institutions that are prevalent in each social context. The concept of institutions put forth by Saris here is a courageous attempt to encompass the prevalent sociocultural milieu. He defines institutions:

> ...as bundles of technologies, narrative styles, modes of discourse, and as importantly, erasures and silences. Culturally and historically situated subjects produce and reproduce these knowledge, practices and silences as a condition of being within the orbit of the institution. (*ibid.* 42)

He furthers his description by elaborating on *institutions* as helping to constitute stories as well as being sites of narrative production, thereby problematising the relationship between *experience* and the development of the story about that experience (*narrative*) in such a way as to focus the analyst's attention on the specific circumstances of the social field in which narratives are developed and deployed. Moreover, narratives as text would ensure a *thick description* that would demonstrate a better picture of the social context in which the narrative is embedded (*ibid.*). The engagement of narrative in institutions can be approached in at least two ways: first, how the members and non-members of the institutions use narrative in their day-to-day routine activities, and second (emerging from the first), in the ways by which these narratives reproduce or challenge the power structures of the institutions (Linde 2003).

Unlike the usually followed clock time or serial time, where one event comes after another, narratives follow narrative time where the time itself is dependent on the events, explained with a beginning, middle, and end (plots). Mattingly (1994: 812) used the concept of *narrative time* and *emplotment* in the analysis of clinical interactions. For her, *emplotment involves making a configuration in time, creating a whole out of a succession of events (plots)* (ibid.). She elaborates that producing narratives and particularly, the work to create a plot out of a succession of actions, is of direct concern to the actor in the midst of action. Narrative analysis used in clinical interactions generates sufficient space for adequate understanding of the actors' (doctors and patients) perspective about the illness as well as their future plans for the same. According to Mattingly (1994: 821),

> A narrative analysis offers a way to examine clinical life as a series of existential negotiations between clinicians and patients, ones that concern the meaning of illness, the place of therapy within an unfolding illness story, and the meaning of a life which must be remade in the face of serious illness.

It is this perspective of narrative—where narrative is shaped by the *institutions*—that is used to analyse doctor–patient interaction in the context of fever care rendered by allopathic hospitals in the state of Kerala.

6.6 Narrative as a Mode of Communication: Voices of Interaction

In order to contextualise the doctor–patient interaction using narrative analysis, Mishler's (2005: 320) the concept of *voice* is used to analyse these interactions. He argues that,

> Voice represents a particular assumption about the relationship between appearance, reality, and language or, more generally, a "voice" represents a specific normative order. Some discourses are closed and continually reaffirm a single normative order; others are open and include different voices, one of which may interrupt another thus leading to the possibility of a new "order".

Thus, it has to be understood that the idea of voice does not equate with a speaker. One speaker may articulate more than one voice; different speakers may share the same voice. Different voices distinguish contrasting orientations to the world and to the moral order, as each voice realises a particular relationship between the speaker and the world. For Mishler (2005: 321), in clinical interaction, two different voices representing different normative orders were identified: the *voice of medicine* and the *voice of the lifeworld*. He argues further that the voice of medicine dominates the voice of the lifeworld in the medical interview where the patients who occasionally articulate the voice of the lifeworld (based on their personal experiences and pre-occupations) get overlooked by the voice of medicine. The whole clinical interaction then is seen as a struggle for dominance, the voice of the lifeworld occasionally interrupting the voice of medicine (Mishler 2005). The above approach of voice situates the clinical interaction as a dynamic one where the power of the patient is also acknowledged by locating both the patient and the doctor within their sociocultural context. Similar to the above argument, Saris demonstrates (1995) via the narrative of a person diagnosed with schizophrenia how, at several junctures, the *institutions* of medicine and their categories lack insight to understand and tackle the problems faced by the person due to the illness. He also demonstrates how the institutionalised authority of professional expertise reflected in the power to *name* thereby silences and erases other experiences and knowledge. The above approaches based on discourse analysis portray the doctor–patient interaction as an everyday activity of human beings whose meaning becomes obvious through contextual analysis.

6.7 Voice(s) of Medicine

The above perspective is, however, limited by dichotomising the character of the clinical encounter to only two voices, where the voice of medicine is itself seen as homogeneous. Atkinson (1995: 130–142) in his study among haematologists demonstrates how different voices within medicine are articulated and how they can be in conflict with each other. This he elaborates by explaining that the voice of medicine constitutes the voice of experience and the voice of science. He explains the *voice of experience* as one of accumulated experiences and a biographical warrant for knowledge and opinion. By *voice of science*, he means an articulation of knowledge warranted by an appeal to research, viz., published scientific papers as well as textual knowledge. It is obvious that a clinic is a place with a specific purpose, where the voices articulated by the patient will largely be illness-related or those which aid illness expression.

Thus, based on Atkinson's and Mishler's insights on clinical encounter, I would like to argue that it is the voice of illness that will be heard. This obviously would be based on past experiences, perceptions, and worldview (lifeworld). In a medicalised society, it is possible that the voice of illness itself will be *medicalised,* thereby articulating a *medicalised voice of illness*. Thus, there can be different voices that are in constant interaction during a doctor–patient interaction. They are the voice of experience and the voice of science together constituting the *voice of medicine,* owing to Atkinson, and the *medicalised voice of illness* and *lifeworld voice of illness,* together constituting the voice of illness as introduced by Mishler. Thus, for the analysis of doctor–patient interaction in fever care in Kerala, the following model involving voices of illness and voices of medicine will be used. The **voices of illness** are further divided into *lifeworld voice of illness* and *medicalised voice of illness* while **voices of medicine** are divided into *voice of science* and *voice of experience*. During clinical interactions, most of these voices get articulated. An analysis of these will be carried out below, as these voices do have a bearing not only on the prevalent discourse but also on the process of medical care. The above voices in themselves should not be seen as all encompassing, as there can be several other voices that may not fit in any of the above categories. Moreover, the dynamics of these various voices again depend on the context of interaction as well as the actors involved.

6.8   The Context

The present chapter focusses on the interaction between the doctor and the patient during fever care based on the data generated through participant observation. To collect the data, the procedures involved in fever care were observed closely and the events of medical care were recorded (ethnography of the clinic) from the hospitals. In addition, several semi-structured interviews were carried out as clarifications from doctors, patients, and other actors involved in the events. Moreover, the doctor–patient interaction during the clinical encounter was captured on the spot for a few cases, giving due consideration to the context of interactions. This was later used as a text for analysing doctor–patient interactions and was subjected to *narrative analysis* (Czarniawska 2004). Here, the process of clinical decision-making as well as the response of the patient was examined within the context and also in terms of its influence on the outcome of fever care. Above all, follow-up of each case identified at the hospital was also done using a household survey. The data was collected in the local language (Malayalam) and translated to English, keeping in mind the original twists, turns, and the context of the original event. Analysis was done in the first stage using a holistic-content approach as mentioned by Lieblich et al. (1998) and later for each case using Heritage's (2004) approach of identifying institutions in interactions. Though institutions were identified almost 'everywhere' in the interactions, they become most obvious from the turns, sequences, and lexical choices, and more importantly, in the epistemological and other forms of asymmetry (ibid.).

The description about the two hospitals at this juncture is inevitable, as making explicit the settings of the field is the only way by which credibility of anthropological studies can be achieved (Sanjek 1990). **Immanuel Hospital** is a private hospital having bed strength of more than 300 with emergency facilities and laboratory facilities capable of doing usual biochemical tests. The hospital offers specialisation for general medicine, paediatrics, ENT, ophthalmology, orthopaedic, skin and VD, and others. Usually, three physicians consult patients at three sites within the general medicine department every day in the hospital. The **Community Health Centre** is a hospital that acts as a primary-level facility within the government sector, a recently upgraded one, where 16 beds are available for inpatients. The centre implements and monitors public health activities (communicable disease control, health education, etc.) in the area. As the hospital is responsible for community level control programmes like TB, malaria, filariasis, and blindness control programmes, the laboratory offers facilities only for sputum tests for TB, blood smear tests for malaria and filariasis, urine tests for diabetes, and eye testing. The additional details of the above hospital settings that were discussed in the first chapter help to build an understanding of the medical care scenario prevalent in the community and thus an understanding of the context of doctor–patient interactions that take place there. Of the three cases used in this chapter, the first two were collected from Immanuel Hospital from two different physicians and a third one was from the CHC.

6.9 Voice of Illness

Jincy Joseph, a 17-year-old girl studying in class XI, went to a practitioner at Immanuel Hospital accompanied by her mother and a neighbour. She reported body pain, fever, and headache. She belongs to a middle-class family for which her brother, working in the military service, is the major source of income. Her parents are educated to the tenth-grade standard and run a small *pettikada* (a small shop-like structure where lemon juice, some sweets, soda, chewing items, cigarettes, etc. are sold). The physician she consulted with completed his medical degree from one of the leading medical colleges of the country and did his post-graduate studies in general medicine. He has been practising since 1972 and has been the physician of this particular hospital for the last eight years.

After completing the registration procedures of the hospital, the patient along with her mother and neighbour entered the consulting room to meet with the physician. Their interaction was as follows [D, doctor (physician); P, patient; MoP, mother of the patient]:

1 D: What is your illness?
P: Fever, severe pain in the legs.
1 MoP: Severe weakness and headache.
2 D: Was there *swelling*? (*Swelling* used in English).

2 MoP: She is very weak, and at times, there is swelling on the side of the feet. Sometimes there is difficulty in breathing and back pain, especially after coming back from the school... she has to walk long distance... she gets very tired.

3 D: Is it hereditary?

3 MoP: No.

4 D: Show your tongue, open your mouth. Is there recurrent throat pain or any other illness?

P: (opening mouth) Ah! No.

(The doctor performed a physical examination by examining the patient's mouth, palpating her abdomen, and listening to her lungs, and then prescribed an echocardiogram (ECG), and routine[1] blood and urine tests.)

MoP: What is the disease, Doctor?

D: I need to see whether it is the initial stages of *arthritis*. Anyway, let me have a look at the test results (*arthritis* used in English).

The doctor then asked the patient to return the next day.

On the second day, after checking the lab test results, the doctor said: '[The] lab test results are normal and the illness could be due to excess strain due to traveling. Medicines for swelling and weakness are written'.

When the consultation ended, the patient collected the medicines from the pharmacy and left to go home. Later, upon examining the medical case record, it was found that neither a diagnosis nor any symptoms were written on the case record, unlike in other cases where at least the symptoms were written. All the lab test results were within the normal ranges. The names of the medicines (Valz, Radiplex, and Complet) prescribed were also written on the case record. Later, during the follow-up of the patient at her home one month after discharge, it was found that she continued to suffer from the illness. Moreover, it was discovered that before coming to the hospital, she tried using steam inhalation at her home to treat the illness and thereafter visited a small clinic nearby that prescribed a *tonic* (a kind of syrup usually taken to resist weakness and enhance health, whose name the patient did not remember). This clinic was run by a qualified allopathic doctor and had no facility for inpatient care but did have basic laboratory facilities. When the illness did not subside, the patient sought care from the Immanuel Hospital.

---

[1]Based on the discussion with laboratory staff of private hospitals and medical college hospital laboratories, it was found that for any disease with fever as the symptom, a *routine blood and urine test* comprised of the following are prescribed: Albumin and bile pigment is looked for in urine and blood, ESR, WBC count [total and differential count (TLC, DLC)], platelet count, urea level, serum bilirubin, serum amylase and creatinine phosphokinase (CPK). None of these indicate the direct presence or absence of any bacteria or virus, rather they are an indication of the physiological functioning of human organs (systems), viz., the liver and kidney, and therefore are also known as liver and kidney function tests. These tests are usually carried out to aid the nature and type of treatment rendered.

During my conversation with the mother about the illness of her daughter, she said that,

> … [she] complains of weakness every day and invariably goes to sleep as soon as she comes home from school. She is not able to study properly. She doesn't help me in any household work. She is very lazy and she complains of weakness … as the illness was not subsiding and news of epidemic diseases made us think that the illness could be serious, we decided to do a complete check-up in the highly reputed private hospital.

The patient's complaints in the above case were similar to those of 'kkk' syndrome,[2] because of which she was unable to study as well as to perform daily household duties. During the clinical interaction, it was obvious that this problem was not addressed adequately. Instead, the search for symptoms by the physician dominated the interaction, as revealed by his question (2 D). It should be noted that despite the expression of the problem by the mother (2 MoP) based on her experience of her daughter's suffering, this information was discounted by the subsequent direct question of the physician (3 D) on heredity. Thereafter, the physical examination portrayed how the voice of medicine dominates the lifeworld voice of illness during the clinical interaction. It appears that the major purpose of the physician's consultation was to collect information regarding *medically-acceptable illnesses*. In other words, the mother of the patient presents the illness in terms of abnormality of the *social body* by demonstrating her daughter's problem as an inability to perform daily chores, travel to school, study her lessons, and help in household work (2 MoP). In contrast, the physician first enquires about heredity to find some clue (3 D) on the abnormality of the *physical body* (physiology), reflected in the physical examination (4 D), and later via the use of technological aid (5 D) for diagnosis. This leads to a one-sided interaction where the patient becomes a mere object in the whole process of therapeutic care. It is interesting to note that the use of the term *swelling* and *arthritis* in the English language, despite having simple, popular translations in Malayalam (*neeru* and *vaatham),* also shows the intense urge of the physician to transform the patient's complaints from *lay* (problems) into textual medical categories. In other words, this was the moment at which the translation of lay category to medical categories took place, whether it represented a symptom (swelling) or a suspected disease (possibility of arthritis).

The above case also demonstrates the management of *uncertainty* during clinical interactions where no valid diagnosis or any symptoms were identified: despite the lack of clarity, medicines were still prescribed. This uncertainty was illustrated in the shifts from the doctor's initial expectation of a possible hereditary factor (3 D) to the possibility of arthritis (5 D) before seeing the lab results. Later, the concluding statement refers only to swelling and weakness, which essentially left the diagnosis at the symptom level. Atkinson (1995: 113–117) in his study among haematologists demonstrated how uncertainty has become an important

---

[2]The term 'kkk' syndrome was coined by general practitioners in South India and stands for 'kai kaal kodachal' (in Tamil), meaning weakness of hands and legs, for which the medical reasons are often unknown.

characteristic of contemporary biomedicine. He elaborated upon the relevance of close examination in the process of everyday medical work as follows:

> It is necessary to pay rather close attention to how uncertainty or certainty are actually conveyed in the course of everyday medical work…There is need for detailed examination of how medical practitioners, students, scientists and others express and discuss their information, how they voice their opinion and how they claim particular warrants for the knowledge and interpretations they endorse (ibid. 17).

He cautions the need to examine and understand the context of uncertainty or certainty and how these are accomplished in everyday medical work. The implications of the outcome become a matter of the power–knowledge relationship that is prevalent in a society. Fox (2000) examines how doctors get socialised through their medical training to manage uncertainties at various levels of medical care, thereby internalising this *ability* as an achieved quality of the art.

6.10 Medicalised Voice and Voice(s) of Medicine

Ramachandran, a 31-year-old married man and a commerce graduate working in a private finance company, went to a private hospital with complaints of fever and body pain. He belongs to a middle-class extended family comprised of his parents, two younger brothers, and a younger sister. The hospital where he sought treatment was the Immanuel Hospital mentioned earlier. The physician he consulted was a younger one, around 36 years old, with a medical degree as well as a post-graduate degree in general medicine. The physician has been practising for eight years, of which seven years were in the above-mentioned hospital. The doctor–patient interaction during consultation was as follows:

1 D: Uh, what is the problem?
1 P: Fever and body pain.
2 D: For how many days?
2 P: Around two to three days.
3 D: Was there vomiting present?
3 P: No, there are rashes in my body.
4 D: Take off your shirt and turn around (Ramachandran's body was full of rashes.).
[Investigations were carried out by the physician using a stethoscope. He later examined the patient's mouth using a tongue depressor.]
4 P: (While examination was going on): I have been taking medicine for jaundice. My serum bilirubin was tested from a nearby lab and the value was 1.1.
5 D: Have you heard of measles?
5 P: No.

6 D: It is a viral infection, and the typical clinical symptoms are shown (*'Viral infection'* and *'typical clinical symptoms'* spoken in English).
7 D: You are getting admitted, aren't you?
6 P: Yes.

When the patient was admitted, routine blood tests were initially carried out. The platelet count was tested daily until the third day, when the patient was discharged from the hospital. At the time of discharge, medicine was prescribed for one more week. The patient was relieved of the illness only ten days after being discharged. Per the medical record, the diagnosis was '?Measles with URTI', indicating that the physician suspected the patient was suffering from measles with an upper respiratory tract infection. On talking with the physician about fever care later, especially regarding the need for laboratory tests in diagnosing the patient, he opined that 'all fever except viral fever need basic laboratory parameter support'. He also added when asked about the platelet count and its relevance that 'unless and until platelet count becomes normal, we cannot discharge a patient'. Later during follow-up at the patient's residence, he commented about his illness:

> … as there was discoloration in urine together with body pain and rashes in the body, I checked serum bilirubin from a nearby lab and as the value was higher than the normal, I went to the hospital.

In the above interaction after the initial problem identification session, the physician's need to make decisions based upon *medically relevant information* becomes clear, as this need ignored the patient's suspicion (4 P) of jaundice. The way the physician assured/justified his finding to himself is visible in his use of terms like *viral infection, typical clinical symptoms* in English (6 D). These are the textual terms that shape the physician's *thought style* or *clinical mentality*. It appears that in a place where English is not the mother tongue, the use of English for unusual terminology during clinical interaction has to be seen as the point at which the translation of clinical presentations (patient's illness) to textual knowledge (medical categories) occurs.[3] The moment in which the patient felt that the examination was over and before the doctor reached a conclusion, the patient offered his own analysis about the illness by pointing to the fact that he was taking medicine for jaundice and that his blood test showed an abnormal value (4 P). Here, the fact that the patient associates serum bilirubin and its elevated value with jaundice, which is logically possible, is a way of expressing his illness in medical terms. In other words, this is the *medicalised voice of illness* that can be heard in many clinical interactions. This medicalised voice may not always be correct, though it was in this case where the

---

[3]It should be noted that only a few terms were used in English during the whole clinical interaction. With the medium of his medical education being in English, it is possible that the physician had internalised certain medical categories and terminology in English only where their translation to the local language (Malayalam) might not be necessary; this is reflected in his use of those terms during clinical interactions.

patient associated serum bilirubin with jaundice. The response of the physician may be either acceptance or rejection. In this instance, it is clear that the physician rejected the medicalised voice of the patient and supplanted it with his authoritative *voice of medicine*—using a *clinical* diagnosis to overrule the serum bilirubin lab values. This occurred despite the fact that the physician seemed to be dependent on laboratory tests for clinical diagnosis as well as for fever care, as reflected in his response to follow-up questions shown above.

The prevalent threat of dengue fever in the society might have possibly influenced the doctor in suspecting dengue fever as a diagnosis, as reflected in his advice for admission as well as checking platelet count every day until the day of discharge from the hospital. This is because cases of measles are not normally admitted, and platelet count—which has nothing to do with measles—is used extensively by the private hospitals as a test for dengue fever. In other words, the above case also demonstrates how during epidemics, *threat* and *medicalisation* influence each other, forming a vicious cycle that further aggravates the process of medicalisation.

This medicalised voice of illness has to be seen as an outcome of the patients' past experiences with illness and the Western medical system, resulting in a state which Crawford (1980: 373) called *healthism and medicalisation of everyday life*. He argues that:

> Past therapeutic experiences and notions derived from diffused medical ideas as well as reinforcing ideological premises of the society acquired by other means pre-structure the encounter *(therapeutic)*. The client *(patient)* is already, in a sense 'professionalised'. In other words, persons being helped take on as their own some of their helpers' theorised assumptions and explanations.

In the above case, the medicalised voice of illness was heard. This demonstrates the above argument that the context of the patient offers a 'professionalised' outlook about his illness as well as everyday life. A similar but different phenomenon that occurs during clinical interaction is the genesis of new categories. This is demonstrated in the following case.

6.11 Therapeutic Interaction: A Site of Knowledge Production

Saritha, a 21-year-old woman, presented to the CHC with fever, headache, and weakness. Her father accompanied her. Her family belongs to a lower income group in which her parents are daily-wage labourers. The family is an extended one with two elder brothers, the eldest married with two children. All of them stay together in a small house located on four cents of land. Saritha is occasionally employed by the cashew factory, depending on the availability of work. At the CHC hospital they went to, most common laboratory tests must be carried out at private laboratories situated on the premises. As there is overcrowding in the hospital, the duration of interaction was minimal. The physician was 52 years old, with a basic medical degree and specialisation in child health, and had been practising for 25 years. The interaction between the doctor and the patient was as follows:

1 D: What is the matter?
1 P: Fever, headache, and weakness in hands and feet.
2 D: For how long?
2 P: One week. Everybody in the house has this.
3 D: *Vishapani* (poisonous fever) is there, could be that, it is better to get admitted.

After getting lab tests done, the patient was admitted for four days and eventually discharged after being prescribed medicines for an additional week. Per the doctor, the illness diagnosis was *viral fever*.

The purpose of the above case is to demonstrate how certain kinds of information during doctor–patient interactions get internalised by the patient and how such information later forms a new category for the public. This was clear when the patient said during the follow-up visit at her home, 'The illness was *vishapani*. This is not like earlier ones. There is something poisonous that enters the body. That is why this is very severe'. The doctor's version of the story, explained during a later interview, completes the picture. His explanation was:

> … it is just viral fever. Since the patients won't understand it if we say 'viral', it is convenient if we use '*visham*' (poison) instead of viral, as the virus when it enters the body becomes poisonous.

The fact that this was indeed a physician-created category, created ostensibly for patients who may not understand, was illustrated by a number of other patients using the same category of *vishapani* to express their illness. One of the patients, who himself considered his illness as *vishapani* when asked about it, responded by saying: 'last time I came with symptoms of fever and body pain, then the doctor said that this is *vishapani*—a new type of fever with severe symptoms'. Here, it is obvious that the context of the doctor–patient interaction becomes a site of knowledge production, knowledge that can determine patient understanding and therefore patient behaviour during illness.

6.12 Interaction of *Thought Styles*

This chapter interprets the doctor–patient interaction during fever care in the state of Kerala where recurrent epidemics were reported. The durations of the interactions were very short, as the study was carried out on presentations of an acute illness like fever and also in local health institutions. The study showed how fear of epidemics generated a perceived *threat* among the public about fevers that was an outcome of the media reports as well as several *control programmes* initiated in the state. In the case of Jincy, the problem the patient put forth was a *social one*, in which she and her mother tried to present the problem as an inability to perform activities of everyday life. On the contrary, the doctor keenly searched for *medically valid findings* that had physiological explanations. These two different notions about the same event are in fact the reflection of each actor's lived experience and the respective roles they perform. In these interactions, the doctor's aim is to settle the issue by a diagnostic and prescriptive act whereas the patient's purpose is to seek relief. Here, *institutions* manifest in diverse ways in all three cases. In the first, the *threat* of fever was a guiding force in the patient's understanding of the illness, as reflected in the patient's effort to seek treatment. In the *second* case, Ramachandran articulated the *medicalised voice of illness* as the patient's dependence on biomedicine in general, and medical technology in particular, that ultimately reached a state of communicating illness in a language close to medicine. This Giddens [(1990) cf. Rochel de Camargo (2002: 830)] describes as:

> ... how lay people rely on expert systems in everyday life, meaning the myriad of technologies that we interact with on a daily basis without really having a firm grasp on how they work.

Here, the institutions with which the patients engages, be them health institutions, the dominant discourse about fever in society, as well as one's own experience with illness, together constitute an important role in the patient's understanding about health, illness, and cure. This becomes obvious from the *third* case, where new knowledge (the category of *vishapani*) is produced in a clinical setting that is neither medical nor lay knowledge. Each interaction is unique by itself, but the meaning of the illness/disease and therefore the outcome is determined depending on the institutions prevalent within the context that clinical interactions occur and among the actors involved.

The above cases provide a picture of how clinical interaction takes place in a South Indian setting and how these interactions are outcomes of the socialisation of the actors involved, which significantly contribute to the overall medical care. Thus, one can argue that clinical interaction is not merely the two-way communication desired for an exchange of information. Instead, it is the product of the networks through which those actors involved are communicating. In other words, the interactions are the outcome of the influence or socialisation of doctors and patients in their respective contexts. This is similar to the notion of *thought style* by Fleck [(1979) cf. Rochel de Camargo 2002] in the case of physicians, and *lifeworlds* (Mishler 2005) in the case of patients. It is in this context that the interactions between doctors and patients become the interaction of various voices, where voices themselves are representations of illness from various realms. Kirmayer (2000: 169) deals with the real complexity of this interaction when he says that,

> Doctor and patient are attempting to communicate, but their conversation is heavily constrained by the demands of the situation and their efforts to present an appropriate face to each other. Each speaks from a different position, which includes awareness of both the interactional context and its relationship to larger social spheres. Each speaks with the voice of the self but invokes the voice of others.

References

Advani, M. (1980). *Doctor patient relationship in Indian hospitals.* Jaipur, India: Sanghi Prakashan.

Atkinson, P. (1995). *Medical talk and medical work: The liturgy of the clinic.* London: Sage Publications.

Crawford, R. (1980). Healthism and medicalisation of everyday life. *International Journal of Health Services, 10*(3), 365–388.

Czarniawska, B. (2004). *Narratives in social science research.* London: Sage.

Emanuel, J. E., & Emanuel, L. L. (1992). Four models of the physician-patient relationship. *Journal of American Medical Association, 27*(16), 2221–2226.

Fleck, L. (1979). *Genesis and development of a scientific fact.* Chicago: University of Chicago Press.

Fox, R. C. (1957). Training for Uncertainty. In R. K. Merton, G. R. George, & P. L. Kendall (Eds.), *The student physician* (pp. 204–241). Cambridge, MA: Harvard University Press.

Fox, R. C. (2000). Medical uncertainty revisited. In L. A. Gary, R. Fitzptrick, & S. C. Scrimshaw (Eds.) *Handbook of social studies in health and medicine,* London: Sage.

Frank, A. (1995). *The wounded storyteller: Body, illness and ethics.* Chicago: University of Chicago Press.

Friedson, E. (1970). *The professions of medicine: A study of the sociology of applied knowledge.* Dodd, New York: Mead.

Friedson, E. (2001, 1970). The profession of medicine. In M. Purdy, & D. Banks (Eds.), *The sociology and politics of health: A reader* (pp. 130–134) London: Routledge.

Giddens, A. (1990). *The consequences of modernity.* London: Polity Press/Basil Blackwell.

Good, B. J., & Good, M. D. (2000). Clinical narratives and the contemporary doctor-patient relationships. In G. Albrecht, R. Fitzpatrick, & S. Schrimshaw (Eds.) *Handbook of social studies in health and medicine.* London: Sage.

Heritage, J. (2004). Conversation analysis and institutional talk: Analysing data. In D. Silverman (Ed.), *Qualitative research: Theory method and practice* (2nd ed.). London: Sage.

Kirmayer, L. J. (2000). Broken narratives clinical encounters and the poetics of illness experience. In M. Cheryl & C. G. Linda (Eds.), *Narrative and the cultural construction of illness and healing.* Berkeley: University of California Press.

Lieblich, A., Tuval-Mashaich, R., & Zilber, T. (1998). *Narrative research: Reading, analysis, and interpretation.* Thousand oaks: Sage.

Linde, C. (2003). Narratives in institutions. In D. Schiffrin, D. Tannen, & H. Hamilton (Eds.) *Handbook of discourse analysis* (pp. 518–536). New York: Blackwell Publishers.

Mattingly, C. (1994). The concept of therapeutic 'emplotment'. *Social Science and Medicine, 38*(6), 811–822.

Mattingly, C., & Garro, L. C. (1994). Introduction: Narrative representations of illness and healing. *Social Science and Medicine, 38*(6), 771–774.

Mattingly, C., & Garro, L. C. (2000). Narrative as construct and construction. In M. Cheryl & C.G. Linda (Eds.), *Narrative and the cultural construction of illness and healing.* Berkeley: University of California Press.

McCormick, J. S. (1979). *The doctor: Father figure or plumber.* London: Croom Helm.

Mechanic, D. (1976). *The growth of bureaucratic medicine: An inquiry into the dynamics of patient behaviour and the organisation of medical care.* New York: John Wiley and Sons.

Mishler, E. G. (2005). The struggle between the voice of medicine and the voice of lifeworld. In P. Conrad (Ed.), *The sociology of health and illness, critical perspectives* (17th ed.). United Kingdom: Worth Publishers.

Moen, T. (2006). Reflections on the narrative research approach. *International Journal of Qualitative methods, 5*(4), 56–69.

Parsons, T. (1951). *The social system.* London: Routledge and Kegan Paul.

Rochel de Camargo, K. (2002). The thought style of physicians: Strategies for keeping up with medical knowledge. *Social Studies of Science, 32*(5–6), 827–855.

Sanjek, R. (1990). On ethnographic validity. In R. Sanjek (Ed.), *The fieldnotes, makings of anthropology*. Ithaca and London: Cornell University Press.

Saris, J. A. (1995). Telling stories: Life histories. *Illness Narratives and InstitutionalLandscapes, Culture, Medicine and Psychiatry, 19*, 39–72.

Seal, S. C. (1971). *An Introduction to hospital-patient relationship*. Kolkata: Nababharat Publishers.

Tuckett, D. (1976). Doctors and patients. In D. Tuckett (Ed.), *An introduction to medical sociology*. London: Tavistock.

Waitzkin, H. (1979). Medicine, Superstructure and Micropolitics. *Social Science and Medicine, 13A*, 601–619.

Chapter 7
Fever Talk as a Sub-culture of Fever Care

This book is about fever talk and fever care. Fever, a very common illness, has had its meaning transformed throughout history and also during various stages of the disease, thus unravelling the complexities around it. The understandings of what constitute fever as an experienced illness, which range from elevated body temperature to runny nose, weakness, and so on, often manifest as a perception of serious threat during the initial stages of the illness, with many patients fearing that it could signal some epidemic disease that can become fatal. This study found that considerably different understandings exist among public health professionals, the media, the public, and the medical fraternity and so on. In the media, sensational headlines are used to create *news*, whereas for the physician, the purpose of utilising different notions of fever is to cure those affected by them. The public's understandings are based on a desired to get rid of both the illness and the threat due to the fear of epidemics. The nature and characteristics of the illness itself are complex, since fever is a major symptom in all the major epidemic diseases noted here—except in the case of leptospirosis—and since all are viral in origin, they follow very similar medical interventions for treatment.

The middle of the 1990s marked the start of fevers being identified as an epidemic because of their increased prevalence as well as the rise in fatalities reported due to specific diseases with fever as a major symptom. Of the several diseases that were reported with fever as symptoms, leptospirosis, dengue fever, viral fevers, and chikungunya struck the hardest and are believed to have resulted in several deaths. This is despite the fact that Japanese encephalitis and malaria were identified in certain pockets during specific seasons. The media fuelled the above scenario by introducing a new category of deaths, *panimaranangal*, meaning death due to fevers, and not only wreaked havoc among the public, but also had the effect of trivialising the distinction between fever as a symptom with other epidemic diseases like leptospirosis, dengue fever, viral fever, and chikungunya. Furthermore, the media followed the biomedical notion of diseases uncritically by using the medical

© Springer Science+Business Media Singapore 2017
M. George, *Institutionalizing Illness Narratives*,
DOI 10.1007/978-981-10-1905-0_7

categories, thereby creating more uncertainty and perception of threat in the community. There were instances when the media also reported those deaths whose causes could not be established by the physicians as fever, further encouraging the fear of fevers.

People began to perceive fevers as well as other epidemic diseases as if both were similar. This tendency reached its peak as the hospitals and the dominant medical system failed to not only follow a uniform disease-definition criterion for each of the epidemic diseases, but also to make a distinction between the two, which ultimately made the understanding of fever very complex. The reporting system prevalent in the state revealed the inadequacy of an efficient reporting system, along with the fact that for a range of fevers, it was found that patients were cured without a final valid diagnosis. This led to a possibility of over-reporting all 'fevers' within one single category to be feared, as if all were communicable fevers (*pakarchapani*) and fever deaths (*panimaranangal*) had become the new threat. An unintended consequence of this was then the under-reporting of diseases like leptospirosis with fever as the major symptom, due to inadequate diagnoses and the poor information systems that existed in the health services system. This societal notion of fevers as a serious threat resulted in the perception of a heightened risk of fevers among lay people, and in turn has had a significant impact on their response towards fevers and therefore on their treatment-seeking behaviour—which, in a highly consumerist state like Kerala, has become medicalised.

For public health professionals, the epidemics of fever were similar to experiences with other epidemics where regular monitoring, surveillance, and early diagnosis and treatment constituted the advice offered, made obvious from the guidelines released during the epidemic. This response was flawed in terms of the insensitivity of the planners towards the actual conditions of the health facilities functioning in the state that were not in a position to follow the recommendations of the guideline. Additionally, of the routine programming that was put forth, comprised of sanitation, health education, and more importantly, the establishment of fever clinics, the former two failed to address the larger issues of development, which in turn needed to address the social determinants of health like environmental and other factors that link health problems to the living and working conditions of those affected. The fever clinics, a new type of medical institution, were started partly as a public health response to the epidemic, but more importantly as a political response to the epidemics. This was obvious from the fact that inadequate planning had gone into the process of establishing the clinics, in which a clear definition on disease categorisation as well as an effective system for monitoring was lacking. Moreover, as mentioned in Chap. 3, the two events that actually ignited the establishment of fever clinics did not have much to do with the then-prevalent epidemics of fever. This inadequacy in planning might have resulted in the setbacks that the new institutions have faced. One of the major setbacks was lack of coordination between the public and private health facilities, as fever clinics were restricted only to the public hospitals in areas with significant utilisation of the private health services, one of the reasons to vouch for a more state-supported health services system. Second, the *fever clinics* and their functions are not immune to the problems faced by the pre-existing outpatient clinics in government hospitals, which are already subjected to several shortcomings including funding cuts, lack of adequate staff, and overcrowding. Failing to address these issues within the health services system makes it difficult to successfully carry forward any new initiative within the public health services, which was later proved true when the fever clinics failed to function as planned.

It is in this context of fever talk that fever care was examined. As historians have always believed that the history of fevers is also the history of medicine, it is true that fever care is a subculture of medical care. Fever clinics, whose major function is fever care, was analysed both as a case of *provisioning* of medical care and as *culture* of medical practice. In Kerala, where the access and utilisation of health services is much greater compared to other states in the country, we found that the time of seeking treatment was influenced by the nature and characteristics of the illness (severity). The nature and characteristics of the fevers studied, indicated by lay interpretation and biomedical interpretation, revealed that the majority of the fevers were not very serious. The multiple interpretations of fevers by the people revealed the role of fear and the contribution of risk perception in people's responses to fever and their implications in public health. This examination involves a kind of 'post-modern' risk, wherein the virtual hazard (epidemic fevers) is projected based on the statistical risk, which will only be validated based on the actual occurrence of events. Any failure to validate the hazard based on the actual occurrence of events (facts or evidence) raises scepticism towards the projected risk. Another dimension to the risk discourse and fear of death was also a reflection of the repeated failure of the state to provide basic services including health care, thereby failing to build the trust of its citizens towards the existing structures of the state; in this light, a form of risk emanated from vulnerability. This heterogeneous notion of risk is helpful in studying how the notions of risk can be different across social groups. The meanings attributed to fever by the people revealed that their understanding is tuned both by their way of life as well as those messages trans-mitted by the dominant biomedical understanding. This lay understanding indicates the complexities involved in the conceptualisation of fever, where every under-standing is rooted in its context and appears to be logical. In other words, the varied notions of fever can be seen to represent an interaction of the varied knowledge systems prevalent in the society, as well as how each of them interact in the process and are in mutual conflict or in concordance. This becomes obvious from the commonalties and differences in the lay and biomedical interpretations of fever, rooted in two different knowledge systems, both influencing each other.

The illness behaviour patterns of patients reveal the extent of dependence on the allopathic system, as reflected by the patients' knowledge about fevers and their self-medication practices. Additionally, the clear shift of the society towards *medicalisation* is indicated by the replacement of home remedies with allopathic medicine. This is also not merely a patient-oriented phenomenon, but one of larger social dynamics reflected in the inevitable role of laboratory investigations in dis-ease diagnosis, an implication of the changing nature of medical practice. Moreover, it is worth mentioning that admission in hospitals is becoming a prerequisite for valid diagnosis, a hospital-specific characteristic that enhances the process of medicalisation and gets intensified by the introduction of insurance in health care, usually denoted by the term 'moral hazard'. The most disturbing part is that despite all these interventions carried out at the hospital, only 14 % of the total cases in our study had a final valid diagnosis, with another 23 % being in the suspected diagnosis category. In other words, around 63 % of the patients were diagnosed only up to the symptom level.

The health services utilisation and health-expenditure patterns of these households indicate that on one hand, the public-sector health services are still a relief for the poor, as reflected in their greater preference of this sector. In societies where access to health services is greater, the time (when) of seeking treatment appears to be more influenced by the nature of illness than by socio-economic conditions. While the choice of health facility (where) is determined primarily based on the economic considerations of the patients, the nature of the illness and the past experiences of the patient with the specific illness and the type of health facility do have considerable influence on the same. Additionally, the major reason for non-treatment of ailments during the early stages of fever was the non-seriousness of the illness. The medical expenditure incurred by patients and its comparison across public and private sectors indicate the commercialisation potential even for a minor illness like fevers. The difference in the expenditure in fever care also reveals the tremendous difference between primary- and secondary-level care within the private sector itself. Further, the overall nature of medical care and, more specifically, the expenditure pattern for fever care also point to the commodification of medical care that exists in the society. This could be an outcome of the providers seeking to raise the existing 'standard' of medical care even for minor illness while capturing the market for health care. 'Raising the standard' is achieved by offering more and more medical interventions than are realistically warranted in medical care. It is important to note that these interventions are not necessarily always scrutinised for actual (rational) need or whether they are commercially driven. This is a unique situation within medical practice, as the onus of this question ultimately lies with the physician and the medical field, keeping it beyond the purview of the lay public who thus remain powerless.

Fever care in this book implies both provisioning as well as the culture of medical practice, as both these mutually influences each other. In other words, provisioning of fever care can be explained and understood only if fever care per se is clearly understood in its complexity. Practising physicians in everyday practice do not necessarily investigate diseases at the cellular level, which can offer a more authentic and valid diagnosis of a disease by identifying the causative agent. Investigating diseases at the cellular (molecular) level require laboratory facilities that need lot of investment to set up, more time (sometimes a week) for the results to arrive, and more importantly, greater costs to be borne by the people. In reality, laboratory investigations at the cellular level hardly take place, not only because they call for better infrastructure and are time consuming and costly for the patients, but also due to the fact that physicians also consider their contribution towards the efficacy of treatment minimal, as treatment is often given in accordance with symptoms. Instead, certain laboratory results that reveal the abnormality of the body, which are usually the *effects* of diseases, are widely used while rendering medical care. For example, the tendency of using lab tests like platelet count and serum bilirubin for diseases like dengue and jaundice, respectively, is a common situation in contemporary medical practice. In other words, those laboratory results like ESR that are not indicative of any specific diseases have, over a period of time, been turned into benchmarks by which healthy and diseased bodies get demarcated. Thus, disease definition virtually depends more on these values wherein the purpose of treatment is to restore these abnormal values instead of to cure the actual illness. Further, these laboratory values, which are merely an indicator of the disease, gradually became the disease-defining criteria as in the case of dengue fever, where platelet count was once an indicator of dengue fever and is now widely used in Kerala and across the country as a test for dengue.

This overdependence on medical technology can result in a medicalised society, as revealed by the tendency of the public to get lab tests done without a doctor's prescription and then present to the hospital with abnormal ESR or serum bilirubin values, without any *visible* somatic illness. This dependence on medical technology —and therefore *normality*—not only side-lines the clinical presentations (illness) that are the starting point of ill health, but an *ideal normal* body based on laboratory values instead becomes the definition of a healthy body. This aspiration of the society to ensure an ideal normal body has also resulted in new avenues for the health care market, especially the field of 'preventive diagnostics', sometimes even projected as a 'public health' intervention by the hospital sector. A close exami-nation of the nature of diagnosis also demonstrates the gaps in the process. These gaps were clear from the fact that the process through which diagnosis happens does not necessarily follow the basic criteria of medical practice, as revealed in the diagnosis of pyrexia of unknown origin (PUO). Moreover, the claim of biomedicine that treatment is for the disease (causative agent) no longer becomes valid, since the uncertainty in medicine often prevents eliciting the causative agent even if one goes to the cellular level, as demonstrated by the cases on treatment modalities. This is obvious in the real-life situations where treatment is rendered in the absence of any valid diagnosis (symptomatic treatment), such as the practice of prescribing antibiotics for viral fever. Besides, in the case of fever care, we observed that the occurrence of a final valid diagnosis became a rarity, and at times the same illness was officially recorded in one way and then communicated differently to the patient. Here, it is worth mentioning that there is inadequate access for the patients to their own medical records in hospitals, and especially in private hospitals. Going further, even when the patients have access they may not be able to interpret the medical record, as the language used in a case record becomes intelligible only to the medical fraternity. In public hospitals, patients have greater access to medical files, however, only minimal information is depicted in the medical record and a majority of the patients belong to a lower socio-economic class and are less educated. On the contrary, in private hospitals the description in the medical record tends to be more detailed but the access to the record is then the most limited because of a greater *sacredness* attached to this information. The benefits of dual reporting for private hospitals could be to accomplish greater popularity through promotion of the idea that the hospital is capable of treating an epidemic disease of greater severity, which ensures greater number of patients and therefore more profits. Moreover, this kind of dual diagnosis helps to conceal medical uncertainty to some extent, thereby legitimising the gaps within medical practice.

This happens because of a lack of uniform disease definition, the absence of a final disease diagnosis, the dependence on a particular kind of medical technology and laboratory techniques, and lastly, reliance on symptomatic treatment are all features of contemporary medical care in the state and are also the case with fever care. These were demonstrated in our analysis of the culture of fever care. As these are features of both public and private hospitals, it can be argued that they constitute the outcome of the nature and characteristics of biomedicine per se. These gaps in the practice of medicine are utilised by market forces, a feature reflected in the greater cost of care in private hospitals as well as the changing nature of hospitals. This is reflected in the fact that hospital admission has become a criterion for diagnosis and patients with insurance coverage increasingly demand admission. In other words, the very nature and characteristics of biomedicine provide space for the market forces to interfere and exert their power on the beneficiaries. This exertion of power reaches its peak through propagation of the popular notion of biomedicine: that it has the ability to solve all health problems and is a practice based on a theoretical understanding of physiology and pathology, as claimed by the allopathic medical fraternity. Furthermore, the inadequate planning that allowed the establishment of fever clinics as part of the state's public health services also resulted in aggravating the faulty notion that medical care alone can ensure population health. In fact, medicine can only render *care,* while the extent of a *cure* that it can offer for a range of diseases is still a debatable issue.

The role of health facilities in propagating these notions about health, illness, and cure is obvious from the doctor–patient interaction where two notions about the same event enter into a negotiation that mostly ends with the domination of physician perspective and therefore that of biomedicine. This provides a picture of how clinical interactions take place in a South Indian setting and how these interactions contribute to the overall medical care. Clinical interaction is not merely the two-way communication desired for exchange of information. Instead, it is the product of the networks through which those actors involved are communicating. In other words, the interactions are the outcome of the influence or socialisation of doctors and patients in their respective contexts. This, for the doctor, is based on the socialisation that occurred during medical training whereas for the patient, it is his or her lived experiences that ultimately get articulated as illness.

This dominance of biomedicine and therefore of physicians should be perceived as a reflection of the prevalent notions about health, illness, and cure that exist in the society. The biomedical understanding of illness (symptoms or diseases) gains relevance during the doctor–patient interaction, thereby discounting the patient's lived experience that is rooted in the social context in which it is embedded. It is this conflict of interest between the patient and the physician that most of the time leads to diverse understandings about the same event, and that can hamper the process of medical care. In addition, the interactions also demonstrate the complexity of the doctor–patient interaction, as the influence of institutions becomes obvious in the outcome of medical care.

7.1   Medical Care and Medical Practice

The issues raised in this study might appear to be specific to fever, but in fact they are applicable to biomedicine in general, as fever care is situated within the larger context of medical care. In any examination of medical care, the components of provisioning and the culture of medical practice cannot be seen in isolation, as both factors can influence and even control each other. To elaborate, provisioning is largely a question of allocation of resources and infrastructure that further takes into consideration government policies and political will. The purpose of provisioning is to ensure equitable distribution of medical care, thereby ensuring adequate access for the needy. In the state of Kerala, the goal of ensuring universal care for all, with an emphasis on biomedicine as a panacea for all ills, may have led to a medicalised society whose ill effects are now becoming manifest as problems of medicalisation. In other words, the question arises as to whether it is wise to universalise a system of medicine, which can create dependency and side effects, both at individual and at the societal levels.

Unlike other products that are commodities, the uniqueness of medical care becomes obvious as revealed by its nature and characteristics that have medicalised society by increasing people's dependence on drugs and medical technology. This has occurred despite the fact that biomedicine itself is frequently uncertain with respect to diagnoses and prognoses during fever care. However, on close examination of fever care in both public and private health facilities, certain commonalties like the absence of a final diagnosis, the use of thermometers being substituted by ESR values, and the way diagnoses are arrived at and types of treatment are provided were found to be in contradiction to that envisaged by medical knowledge. Here, the question is whether we attribute these shortcomings to the problems of provisioning of medical care or *whether these are due to the problems of biomedicine* per se *that are being intensified by the problems of provisioning.* I would argue that the latter is true, as the above features are found in both public and private hospitals alike, though their intensity varies.

Moreover, the provisioning of medical care should be in accordance with the understanding of the capabilities and prospects that medicine can offer. The dual power of biomedicine to solve the problems of ill health as well as to exert control on human beings through the act of medical care needs to be acknowledged here. Medicine has ceased to be a subject defined by its explicit and exclusive purpose of healing the sick, and has instead become an applied science, consisting of a pragmatically derived range of disciplines and techniques that claim more and more 'scientificity' and predictability. This has ultimately resulted in further eradicating the personhood of the patient from the medical discourse. The classification of illness has now become a biochemical process or viewed as an outcome of an organic lesion, where analysis and explanation are the occupational task of the medical investigator instead of the previous act of diagnosis and classification that was based more on somatic distress. Thus, on one hand, the changing nature of medicine is such that medical knowledge and medical practice are highly dependent on medical technology and laboratories, thereby narrowing the humanness of medical care and more importantly the social context of the patient. On the other, we have commercial and corporate forces that are hungry to utilise the gaps within medical practice that are internal to the philosophy and logic of medicine, and which become intensified due to medicine's changing nature. It is worth mentioning here that provisioning is not only allocation but also restriction (control) of resources. A realisation of this second aspect needs to be highlighted in the current context of medical uncertainty: in the current scenario, there is wide scepticism of the power of medicine to cure, as well as of its increasing dependence on medical technology and drugs in the process of medical care.

7.2   The Way Forward

The book raises certain issues for discussion. First, upon examining the provisioning of fever care, it was found that contrary to the popular notion that the poor generally utilise public services, some poor patients also use private health facilities in the case of acute illnesses like fever. This was based on rational considerations with economic reasons being the basis, as these patients found private health facilities to be cheaper and provide better services than the public health facility available to them. This occurred in situations where the latter failed to offer its services free of cost, as is generally expected. This calls for the *need to strengthen the public sector with comprehensive services so that the poor will not be burdened,* taking into account the reality where, despite the sector being public, many of the services are actually rendered by the private sector due to inadequate allocation of resources to the former.

The culture of biomedicine demonstrates that there exists a huge difference between the way it is practiced and the way it ought to be. It should be noted that earlier initiatives have attempted to propagate a rational use of drugs and/or rational prescription of laboratory tests, taking into consideration the commodification of medical care. This cannot take us very far, as the irrational practice is only the manifestation of the changing nature and characteristics of biomedicine, whose autonomy lies with the physician. Instead, it would be meaningful to aim at developing a *rational practice of medicine* in which the role of the patient in the whole process of medical care has to be that of an active participant. This should take into consideration the infrastructure facilities available in various health institutions and the social context of the patient, and finally, it should be in tune with the prevalent discourses on health, illness, and cure. This leads to the larger question of medical ethics in terms of how medicine ought to be practised in various settings. This can provide ample scope for the analysis of other systems of medicine as well, where biomedicine and its thought style should be regarded as only one way of seeing the world.

Ultimately, this raises the question of whether we *need to follow a uniform disease definition for each disease, especially during epidemics across allopathic health facilities.* Our case studies showed that varied definitions of the same disease were followed by different allopathic health facilities, with each accusing the other of using invalid definitions. This calls for the need to re-examine the role of disease diagnosis in medical care and to question whether diagnosis is a prerequisite for the practice of medicine or whether it is only the need of the epidemiologist. If diagnosis is required, should it then follow any specific, homogenous, and meaningful criterion, at least within the scholarship of biomedicine?

Glossary

Burdwan fever Another name for kala-azar, as it was found in large numbers in Burdwan in West Bengal

Cent Smallest unit of an acre—100 cents equals one acre

Chikungunya A viral disease caused by the chikungunya virus that was reported in epidemic proportions in various parts of India, especially southern India, in 2006 and 2007

Choodu (*Malayalam*) Literally means heat, used in varied contexts to signify body heat, profuse sweating due to humidity and also to anger

Chukku (*Malayalam*) Dried ginger

Durbar physician Physician in charge of treating the royal family

Jaladoshapani (*Malayalam*) Simple cold fever

Joley cheyyan pattunnilla (*Malayalam*) Unable to do work

Jwar-vikar Another name for kala-azar

Kala-jwar Another name for kala-azar

Kanji (*Malayalam*) A mixture of rice and water prepared by making rice without draining the water

Kashayam (*Malayalam*) A preparation similar to black coffee, in which jaggery, black pepper, and ginger are used

KKK syndrome *kai kaal kodachal*, a Tamil phrase to denote pain in the hands and legs of the patient, the cause of which is unknown—a category widely used among the physicians in south India

Kshinam (*Malayalam*) Weakness of the body

Kurumulakurasam (*Malayalam*) A preparation with tamarind, salt, tomato, pepper, and mustard—a favourite in southern India. During fever, the quantity of pepper will be increased slightly

© Springer Science+Business Media Singapore 2017
M. George, *Institutionalizing Illness Narratives*,
DOI 10.1007/978-981-10-1905-0

Leptospirosis Popularly known as rat fever in Kerala. Also known as Weil's disease, caused by the bacteria *Leptospira*, contracted by humans through the urine and faeces of bandicoot rats

Notifiable disease As part of the surveillance effort, certain diseases treated in the hospital are expected to be reported to the district medical authorities. Inclusion of diseases in the category of *notifiable* diseases is based on the prevalence of certain diseases in epidemic proportions, in order to maintain an effective investigation system

Pani (Malayalam) Widely known as fever. Literal meaning is dew, cool, and is used in various contexts by patients to express body pain, runny nose, cold, cough, and elevated body temperature

Pakarchapani (Malayalam) Meaning attributed to fevers that can be spread (communicable). This is widely used to indicate fevers that can be a symptom for disease epidemics that can be fatal

Panimaranangal (Malayalam) A category used by the media, especially newspapers, to denote deaths happening in the state due to fever

Pettikkada (Malayalam) A small shop-like structure where lemon juice, some sweets, soda, chewing items, cigarettes, etc., are sold, similar to betel-shops in north India

Taluk Small division within a district, specifically with respect to revenue

Thalarcha (Malayalam) Weakness, a kind of fatigue

Vishapani **(Malayalam)** A new term produced during the doctor-patient interaction to indicate viral fever, whose literal translation is poisonous fever

Ward Smallest political division within the panchayats, towns and corporations

Bibliography

Addlakha, R. (2001). State legitimacy and social suffering in a modern epidemic: A case study of dengue haemorrhagic fever in Delhi. *Contributions to Indian Sociology, 35*(2), 151–179.

Advani, M. (1980). *Doctor patient relationship in Indian hospitals*. Jaipur, India: Sanghi Prakashan.

Alonzo, A. A. (1984). An illness behaviour paradigm: A conceptual exploration of a situational adaptation perspective. *Social Science and Medicine, 19*(5), 499–510.

Ananth, M. (2008). *In defense of an evolutionary concept of health: Nature, norms and human biology*. United Kingdom: Ashgate.

Aravindan, K. P. (2006). *Kerala padanam, keralam engane Jeevikkunnu? Keralalm engane chinthikkunnu?(Malayalam): A study on Kerala, how Kerala lives? How Kerala thinks?*. Kozhikode, Kerala: Kerala Sastra Sahitya Parishad.

Armstrong, D. (1995). The rise of surveillance medicine. *Sociology of Health and Illness, 17*(3), 393–404.

Atkinson, P. (1995). *Medical talk and medical work: The liturgy of the clinic*. London: Sage Publications.

Banerji, D. (1989). Rural social transformation and changing health behaviour. *Economic and Political Weekly, 1*, 1474–1480.

Banerji, D. (1984). Breakdown of public health system. *Economic and Political Weekly, 19*(22), 881–882.

Banerji, D. (1985). *Health and family planning services in India, an epidemiological, socio-cultural and political analysis and a perspective*. New Delhi: Lok Paksh.

Banerji, D., & Anderson, S. (1963). A sociological study of the awareness of symptoms suggestive of pulmonary tuberculosis. *Bulletin of the World Health Organisation, 29*(5), 665–683.

Barnes, B. (1974). *Scientific knowledge and sociological theory* . London: Routledge and Kegan Paul.

Baru, R., Qadeer, I., & Priya, R. (2002). *State and private sector in India: Some policy options*. New Delhi: Centre of Social Medicine and Community Health, School of Social Sciences, Jawaharlal Nehru University.

Baru, R. (1998). *Private health care in India: Social characteristics and trends*. New Delhi: Sage.

Bates, D. G. (1981). Thomas Willis and the fevers literature of the nineteenth century. In W. F. Bynum & V. Nutton (Eds.), *Theories of fever from antiquity to enlightenment*. Medical History Supplement No. 1, London: Wellcome Institute for the History of Medicine.

Bennett, P., & Hodgson, R. (1992). Psychology and health promotion. In Robin Bunton & Gordon Macdonald (Eds.), *Health promotion, disciplines and diversity*. London and New York: Routledge.

Berg, M. (2004). Practices of reading and writing: The constitutive role of the patient record in medical work. In A. Ella, M. A. Elston, & L. Prior (Eds.), *Medical work, medical knowledge and health care*. United Kingdom: Blackwell.

Boorse, C. (1976). On the distinction between disease and illness. *Philosophy and Public Affairs,* *5*(1), 49–68.

Brown, M. W. (1985). On defining 'disease'. *The Journal of Medicine and Philosophy, 10,* 311–328.

Brown, P. J., Inhorn, M. C., & Smith, D. J. (1996). Disease, ecology and human behaviour. In Carolyn F. Sargent & Thomas M. Johnson (Eds.), *Medical anthropology: Contemporary theory and method* (revised ed., pp. 183–219). Connecticut, London: Praeger.

Bury, M. (1998) Postmodernity and Health. In G. Scambler & P. Higgs (Eds.), *Modernity medicine and health, medical sociology towards 2000* (pp. 1–28). London and New York: Routledge.

Bynum, W. F. (1981). Cullen and the study of fevers in Britain, 1760–1820. In W. F. Bynum & V. Nutton (Eds.), *Theories of fever from antiquity to enlightenment.*Medical History Supplement No. 1, London: Wellcome Institute for the History of Medicine.

Bynum, W. F., & Nutton, V. (1981). Introduction. In W. F. Bynum & V. Nutton (Eds.), *Theories of fever from antiquity to enlightenment.*, Medical History Supplement No. 1, London: Wellcome Institute for the History of Medicine.

Canguilhem, G. (1991). *On the normal and the pathological.* New York: Zone Books.

Cartwright, F. F. (1977). *A social history of medicine.* London: Longman.

Casper, M. J., & Morrison, D. R. (2010). Medical sociology and technology: Critical engagements. *Journal of Health and Social Behaviour, 51*(1S), S120–S132.

Casper, M., & Berg, M. (1995). Introduction: Constructivist perspectives on medical work: Medical practices and science and technology studies. *Science, Technology and Human Values, special issue, 20*(4), 395–407.

Census of India. (2011). Provisional population totals. Series-33. Kerala. Paper 1 of 2001. Thirvananthapuram, India: Director of Census Operations, Kerala.

Clarke, A. E., Shim, J. K., Mamo, L., Ruth, F., & Fishman, J. R. (2003). Biomedicalization: Technoscientific transformations of Health, Illness, and US Biomedicine. In G. Albrecht, R. Fitzpatrick, & S. Schrimshaw (Eds.), *Handbook of social studies in health and medicine* (pp. 442–445). London: Sage.

Cornad, P. (2007). *The medicalization of society: On the transformation of human condition into treatable disorders.* Baltimore: Johns Hopkins University Press.

Crawford, R. (1980). Healthism and medicalisation of everyday life. *International Journal of Health Services, 10*(3), 365–388.

Cunningham, A. (1981). Sydenham versus Newton: The Edinburgh fever dispute of the 1690s between Andrew Brown and Archibald Picairne. In W. F. Bynum & V. Nutton (Eds.), *Theories of fever from antiquity to enlightenment.* Medical History Supplement No. 1, London: Wellcome Institute for the History of Medicine.

Czarniawska, B. (2004). *Narratives in social science research.* London: Sage.

Dilip, T. R. (2005). Extent of inequity in access to health care services in India. In L. V. Gangoli, R. Duggal, & A. Shukla (Eds.), *Review of health care in India.* CEHAT: Mumbai, India.

Dubos, R. (1959). *Mirage of health, utopias, progress and biological change.* Perennial Library, London: Harper and Row Publishers Ltd.

Ehrenreich, J. (1978). Introduction. In J. Ehrenreich (Ed.), *The cultural crisis of modern medicine* (pp. 1–35). New York: Monthly Review Press.

Ekbal, B. (2000). *People's campaign for decentralised planning and the health sector in Kerala.* Issue paper presented in People's Health Assembly 2000 held in Mexico, pp. 1–7.

Emanuel, J. E., & Emanuel, L. L. (1992). Four models of the physician-patient relationship. *Journal of American Medical Association, 27*(16), 2221–2226.

Engel, G. L. (1977). The need for a new medical model: A challenge for biomedicine. *Science, 196* (4286), 129–136.

Engelhardt, T, Jr. (1976). Ideology and etiology. *The Journal of Medicine and Philosophy, 1*(3), 256–268.

Engelhardt, T, Jr. (1976). Ideology and etiology. *The Journal of Medicine and Philosophy, 1*(3), 256–268.

Fleck, L. (1979). *Genesis and development of a scientific fact*. Chicago: University of Chicago Press.

Fleck, L. (1981 [1935]). On the Question of the Foundation of Medical Knowledge. *Journal of Medicine and Philosophy.* 6 (3): 237-56.

Foucault, M. (1975). *The birth of the clinic: Archaeology of medical perception*. New York and London: Vintage Books.

Fox, N. J. (1999). Post modern reflections on risk, hazards and life choices. In D. Lupton (Ed.), *Risk and socio-cultural theory: New directions and perspectives* (pp. 12–33). Cambridge, UK: Cambridge University Press.

Fox, R. C. (1957). Training for uncertainty. In R. K. Merton, G. G. Reader & P. L. Kendall (Eds), *The student physician* (pp. 204–241). Cambridge, MA: Harvard University Press.

Fox, R. C. (1989). *The sociology of medicine, a participant observer's view*. Engelwood Cliffs, New Jersey: Prentice Hall.

Fox, R. C. (2000). Medical uncertainty revisited. In L. A. Gary, R. Fitzptrick & S. C. Scrimshaw (Eds.), *Handbook of social studies in health and medicine*. London: Sage.

Frank, A. (1995). *The wounded storyteller: Body, illness and ethics*. Chicago: University of Chicago Press.

Franke, R., & Chasin, B. (1991). Kerala State, India: Radical Reform as Development. *Monthly Review, 42*(8), 1–23.

Frankenberg, R. (1981) Allopathic medicine, profession, and capitalist ideology in India. *Social Science and Medicine, 15* A (2), 115–125.

Friedson, E. (1970). *The professions of medicine: A study of the sociology of applied knowledge*. Dodd, New York: Mead.

Friedson, E. (2001 [1970]). The profession of medicine. In M. Purdy & D. Banks (Eds.), *The sociology and politics of health: A reader* (pp. 130–134). London: Routledge.

Gallagher, E. R. (1976). Lines of reconstruction and extension in the Parsonian sociology of illness. *Social Science and Medicine, 10*, 207–218.

George. (2016 forthcoming). Health care norms under universal health care (UHC) for Maharashtra: Relieving illness and ensuring public health. *Journal of Health Management, 18*, 4.

George, M. (2014a). Book review: Mahesh Ananth (2008) In defense of an evolutionary concept of health: Nature, norms and human biology. *Medicine Studies: An International Journal of History, Philosophy, and Ethics of Medicine and Allied Sciences, 4*(4), 113–117.

George, M. (2014b). Heterogeneity in private sector health care and its implications on Urban Poor. *Journal of Health Management, 16*(1), 79–92.

George, M. (2007a). *Interpreting fever talk and fever care in Kerala's socio-cultural context*. Unpublished Ph.D thesis, Centre of Social Medicine and Community Health, School of Social Sciences, Jawaharlal Nehru University, New Delhi.

George, M. (2007b). Socio–economic and cultural dimensions and health seeking behaviour for leptospirosis: A case study of Kerala, *Journal of Health Management, 9*(3), 381–398.

George, M. (2010). Voice of illness and voice of medicine in doctor-patient interaction. *Sociological Bulletin, 59*(2), 159–178.

Gerhardt, U. (1987). Parsons' role theory and health interaction. In G. Scambler (Ed.), *Sociological theory and medical sociology*. London: Routledge.

Gerson (1976) The social character of illness: Deviance or politics, *social science and medicine, 10*, 219–224.

Geyer-Kordesch, J. (1981). Fever and other fundamentals: Dutch and German medical explanations c.1680 to 1730. In W.F. Bynum & V. Nutton (Eds.), *Theories of fever from antiquity to Enlightenment*. Medical History Supplement No. 1, London: Wellcome Institute for the History of Medicine.

Ghosh, I., & Lester, C. (2000). An ethnography of cholera in Calcutta. *Economic and Political Weekly, 35*(8&9), 684–696.

Giddens, A. (1990). *The consequences of modernity*. London: Polity Press/Basil Blackwell.

Good, B. J., & Good, M. D. (2000). Clinical narratives and the contemporary doctor-patient relationships. In G. Albrecht, R. Fitzpatrick & S. Schrimshaw (Eds.), *Handbook of social studies in health and medicine*. London: Sage.

Good, B. J. (1994). *Medicine, rationality and experience, an anthropological experience*. Cambridge: Cambridge University Press.

Government of India. (1946). *Health survey and development committee (Bhore Committee) report* (Vol. I). Delhi: Manager of Publications.

Hampton, J. R., Harrison, M. J. G., Mitchell, J. R. A., Prichard, J. S., & Seymour, C. (1975). Relative Contributions of History-taking, physical examination and laboratory investigation to diagnosis and management of medical outpatients. *British Medical Journal, 2,* 486–489.

Harrison, M. (1994). *Public health in British India: Anglo-Indian preventive medicine 1859-1914*. New Delhi: Cambridge University Press.

Heritage, J. (2004). Conversation analysis and institutional talk: Analysing data. In David Silverman (Ed.), *Qualitative research: Theory method and practice* (2nd ed.). London: Sage.

Illich, I. (1975). *Medical nemesis: The expropriation of medical knowledge*. Calcutta: Calder and Boyars.

Jaggi, O. P. (2000). Medicine in India: Modern period. In D. P. Chattopadhyaya (Ed.), *History of science, philosophy and culture in Indian Civilization* (Vol. IX, part I). PHISPC, New York: Oxford University Press (Chp.7).

Jeffrey, R. (1997). Malayalam: 'The day–to–day social life of the people...'. *Economic and Political Weekly, 32*(1 & 2), 18–21 (4–11 January).

Jewson, N. D. (1976). The disappearance of the sick man from medical cosmology 1770-1870. *Sociology, 10,* 225–244.

Jorgensen, M., & Phillips, L. (2002). *Discourse analysis as theory and method*. London: Sage.

Jutel, A. (2009). Sociology of diagnosis: A preliminary review. *Sociology of Health and Illness, 31* (2), 278–299.

Kalra, N., & Prasittisuk, C. (2004). Sporadic prevalence of DF/DHF in the Nilgiri and Cardamom Hills of Western Ghats in South India: Is it a seeding from sylvatic dengue cycle—A hypothesis. *Dengue Bulletin* (Vol. 28, pp. 44–50). SEAR: WHO.

Kannan, K. P., Thankappan, K. R., Ramankutty, V., & Aravindan, K. P. (1991). *Health and development in rural Kerala*. Thiruvananthapuram, Kerala: Kerala Sastra Sahithya Parishad.

Kannan, K. P. (1999). *Poverty alleviation as advancing basic human capabilities: Kerala's achievements compared*. Thiruvananthapuram, Kerala: Centre For Development Studies.

Kasl, S. V., & Cobb, S. (1966). Health behaviour, illness behaviour, and sick role behaviour. *Archives of Environmental Health, 12,* 246–266.

Kawashima, K. (1998). *Missionaries and a Hindu state: Travancore 1858–1936*. New York: Oxford University Press.

King, L. S. (1982). *Medical thinking. A historical preface* (p. 149). Princeton, New Jersey: Princeton University Press.

Kirmayer, L. J. (2000). Broken narratives clinical encounters and the poetics of illness experience. In M. Cheryl & C. G. Linda (Eds.), *Narrative and the cultural construction of illness and healing*. Berkeley: University of California Press.

Kleinman, A. (1980). *Patients and Healers in the Context of Culture. An exploration of the borderland between anthropology, medicine and psychiatry*. Berkeley: University of California Press.

Kleinman, A. (1986). Concepts and a model for the comparison of medical systems as cultural systems. In C. Currer & M. Stacey (Eds.), *Concepts of health, illness and disease* (pp. 29–47). Oxford: Berg publications Ltd.

Kleinman, A., Eisenberg, L., & Good, B. (1978). Culture, illness and care, clinical lessons form anthropologic and cross-cultural research. *Annals of Internal Medicine, 88,* 251–258.

Kohl, K. S., Marcy, M., Blum, M., Jones, M. C., Dagan, R., Hansen, J., et al. (2004). Fever after immunization: Current concepts and improved future scientific understanding. *Clinical Infectious Diseases, 39*(3), 389–394.

Kollam Corporation. (2007). *Pathaam Panchavalsara Paddathi, vikasenarekha 2002–2007 (Malayalam), Development Report, Tenth Plan.* Kollam, Kerala: Kollam Corporation.

Kooiman, D. (1991). Mass movement, famine and epidemic a study in interrelationship. *Modern Asian Studies, 25*(2), 281–301.

Kraupl Taylor, F. (1980). The concept of disease. *Psychological Medicine, 10,* 419–424.

Krishnaswami, P. (2004). *Morbidity Study—Incidence, prevalence, consequences and associates.* Discussion Paper No. 63, Thiruvananthapuram: Kerala Research Programme on Local Level Development, Centre for Development Studies.

Kroeber, A. (1983). Anthropological and socio-medical health care research in developing countries. *Social Science and Medicine, 17*(3), 147–161.

Kumar, A. (1998). *Medicine and the Raj: British medical policy in India 1835–1911.* New Delhi: Sage publications.

Kunjhikannan, T. P., & Aravindan, K. P. (2000). *Changes in health transition in Kerala, 1987–1997.* Thiruvananthapuram, Kerala: Kerala Research Programme on Local Level Development, Centre for Development Studies.

Kunjhikannan, T. P., & Aravindan, K. P. (2000). *Changes in health transition in Kerala, 1987–1997.* Thiruvananthapuram: Kerala Research Programme on Local Level Development, Centre for Development Studies.

Latour, B., & Woolgar, S. (1986). The laboratory life: The construction of scientific facts. Princeton, New Jersey: Princeton University Press.

Lieblick, A., Tuval-Mashaich, R., & Zilber, T. (1998). *Narrative research: Reading, analysis, and interpretation.* Thousand oaks: Sage.

Linde, C. (2003). Narratives in institutions. In D. Schiffrin, D. Tannen & H. Hamilton (Eds.), *Handbook of discourse analysis* (pp. 518–536). New York: Blackwell Publishers (chp 25).

Lonie, I. M. (1981). Fever pathology in the sixteenth century: Tradition and innovation. In W. F. Bynum & V. Nutton (Eds.), *Theories of fever from antiquity to enlightenment* (pp. 19–44). Medical History Supplement No. 1, London: Wellcome Institute for the History of Medicine.

Loustaunau, M. O., & Sobo, E. J. (1997). *The cultural context of health, illness, and medicine* (pp. 145–162). Westport, CT: Bergin & Garvey.

Löwy, I. (1993). Testing for a sexually transmissable disease 1907–1970: The history of the Wassermann Reaction. In V. Berridge & P. Strong (Eds.), *Aids, and contemporary history* (pp. 74–92). Cambridge: Cambridge University press.

Lupton, D. (1993). Risk as Moral Danger: The social and political functions of risk discourse in public health. *International Journal of Health Services, 23*(3), 425–435.

Lupton, D. (1994). *Medicine as culture: Illness, disease and the body in the western societies.* London: Sage.

Mackowaik, P. A. (1998). Concepts of fever. *Archives of Internal Medicine, 158*(17), 1870–1881.

Mackowiak, P. A., Bartlett, J., Borden, E. C., Goldblum, S. E., Hasday, J. D., Munford, R. S., et al. (1997). Concepts of fever: Recent advances and lingering dogma. *Clinical Infectious Diseases, 25*(1), 119–138.

Mattingly, C. (1994). The concept of therapeutic 'emplotment'. *Social Science and Medicine, 38*(6), 811–822.

Mattingly, C., & Garro, L. C. (1994). Introduction: Narrative representations of illness and healing. *Social Science and Medicine, 38*(6), 771–774.

Mattingly, C., & Garro, L. C. (2000). Narrative as construct and construction. In M. Cheryl & C. G. Linda (Eds.), *Narrative and the cultural construction of illness and healing.* Berkeley: University of California Press.

McCormick, J. S. (1979). *The doctor: Father figure or plumber.* London: Croom Helm.

McCullough, L. (1981). Thought-styles, diagnosis, and concepts of disease: Commentary on Ludwick Fleck. *The Journal of Medicine and Philosophy, 6*, 257–261.

McKinlay, J.B. (1972). Some approaches and problems in the study of the use of services, an overview. *Journal of Health and Social Behaviour, 13*, 115–152.

Mckinlay, J. B., & Stoeckle, J. D. (1988). Corporatizaton and the social transformation of doctoring. *International Journal of Health Services, 18*(2), 191–205.

Mechanic, D. (1969). Illness and cure. In J. Kosa, et al. (Eds.), *Poverty and health—A sociological analysis.* London: Harvard University.

Mechanic, D. (1976). *The growth of bureaucratic medicine: An inquiry into the dynamics of patient behaviour and the organisation of medical care.* New York: Wiley.

Mechanic, D. (1993). Social research in health and the American sociopolitical context: The changing fortunes of medical sociology. *Social Science and Medicine, 36*(2), 95–102.

Mishler, E. G. (2005). The struggle between the voice of medicine and the voice of lifeworld. In Peter Conrad (Ed.), *The sociology of health and illness, critical perspectives* (17th ed.). United Kingdom: Worth Publishers.

Moen, T. (2006). Reflections on the narrative research approach. *International Journal of Qualitative methods, 5*(4), 56–69.

Munson, R. (1981). Why medicine cannot be a science. *The Journal of Medicine and Philosophy, 6*, 183–208.

Murray, C. J., & Chen, L. (1992). Understanding morbidity change. *Population and Development Review, 48*, 481–503.

Naraindas, H. (1996). Poisons. *Putrescence and the weather: A genealogy of the advent of tropical medicine, contributions to Indian sociology, 30*(1), 1–35.

Naraindas, H. (2006). Of spineless babies and folic acid: Evidence and efficacy in biomedicine and ayurvedic medicine. *Social Science and Medicine, 62*(11), 2658–2669.

Navarro, V. (1975). The political economy of medical care, an explanation of the compositions, nature and functions of the present health sector of the United States. *International Journal of Health Services, 5*(1), 65–94.

Navarro, V. (1986). *Crisis, health, and medicine, a social critique.* New York: Tavistock Publications.

NSSO. (2015). *Key indicators of social consumption in India: Health,* (NSSO 71st Round, January–June 2014), p. A8.

NSSO. (1998). *Morbidity and treatment of ailments.* Report no. 441. NSS fifty–second round, July 1995–June 1996. New Delhi: National Sample Survey Organization, Department of Statistics, Government of India.

Osella, F., & Osella, C. (1996). Articulation of physical and social bodies in Kerala. *Contributions to Indian Sociology, 30*(1), 37–68.

Panicker, P. G. K., & Soman, C. R. (1984). *Health status of Kerala: The paradox of economic backwardness and health development.* Thiruvananthapuram, Kerala: Centre for Development Studies.

Panicker, P. G. K. (1999). *Health transition in Kerala.* Discussion Paper No.10, Thiruvananthapuram, Kerala: Kerala Research Programme on Local Level Development, Centre For Development Studies.

Panikkar, K. N. (1992). Indigenous medicine and cultural hegemony: A study of the revitalisation movement in Keralam. *Studies in History, 8*(2), 283–308.

Parsons, T. (1951). *The social system.* London: Routledge and Kegan Paul.

Pellegrino, E. D., & Thomasma, D. (1981). *A philosophical basis of medical practice, toward a philosophy and ethic of the healing professions.* New York and Oxford: Oxford University Press.

Petersdorf, R. G. (1974). Disturbances of Heat Regulation. In M. M. Wintrobe.

Pickstone, J. V. (1992). Dearth, dirt and fever epidemics: Rewriting the history of British 'Public Health'. In Terrence Ranger & Paul Slack (Eds.), *Epidemics and ideas, essays on the historical perception of pestilence* (pp. 1780–1850). Cambridge: Cambridge University Press.

Pillai, R. K., Williams, S. V., Glick, H. A., et al. (2003). Factors affecting decisions to seek treatment for sick children in Kerala, India. *Social Science and Medicine, 57*, 783–790.

Prasad, P. (2000). Health care access and marginalized social spaces, leptospirosis in South Gujarat. *Economic and Political Weekly*, 3688–3694.

Prasad, P. (2005). Narratives of sickness and suffering: A study of malaria in South Gujarat. *Sociological Bulletin, 54*(2), 218–237.

Qadeer, I. (2000). Health care systems in transition III India part I. The Indian experience. *Journal of Public Health Medicine, 22*(1), 25–32.

Ramachandran, C. K. (2000). *Vydhyasamskaram (Malayalam): Medical culture*. Calicut, Kerala: Mathrubhumi Printing and Publishing Company Ltd.

Ramachandran, R. (2006). Virulent outbreak. *Frontline. 23*(20) October 07–20, Available at http://www.frontlineonnet.com/fl2320/stories/20061020004911900.htm. Accessed on May 22, 2010.

Rao, S., Nundy, M., & Singh, A. (2005). Delivery of health services in the private sector, In *Financing and delivery of health care services in India*, National Commission on Macroeconomic Commission and Health, background paper, pp. 89–104.

Ratcliffe, J. (1978). Social justice and the demographic transition: Lessons from India's Kerala State. *International Journal of Health Services, 8*(1), 123–144.

Reiser, J. S. (1978). *Medicine and the reign of technology*. Cambridge, United Kingdom: Cambridge University Press.

Reissman, C. K. (2005). Exporting ethics: A narrative about narrative research in south India. *Health: An Interdisciplinary Journal for the Social Study of Health, Illness and Medicine, 9*(4), 473–490. Sage: London.

Remadevi, S., & Dass, S. (1999). *Environmental factors of malaria persistence: A study at Valiyathura, Thiruvananthapuram City*, Discussion Paper No. 3, Thiruvananthapuram: Kerala Research Programme on Local Level Development, Centre for Development Studies.

Renaud, M. (1978). On the structural constraints to state intervention in health. In J. Ehrenreich (Ed.), *The cultural crisis of modern medicine*. New York and London: Monthly Review Press.

Rochel de Camargo, K. (2002). The thought style of physicians: Strategies for keeping up with medical knowledge. *Social Studies of Science, 32*(5–6), 827–855.

Rosenberg, C. (2002). The tyranny of diagnosis, specific entities and individual experience. *The Millbank Quarterly, 80*(2), 237–260.

Rosenberg, C. E. (1989). Disease in history: Frames and framers. *The Milbank Quarterly, 67*(1), 1–15.

Rosenstock, I. M., & Kirscht, J. P. (1979). Why people seek health care? In G. C. Stone, F. Cohen, N. E. Adler and associates (Eds.), *Health psychology—A hand book, theories, applications and challenges of a psychological approach to the health care system*. San Fransisco: Josey Danys Publication.

Rothstein, G. W. (2003). *Public health and the risk factor: A history of an uneven medical revolution*. USA: University of Rochester Press.

Sagar, A. D. (1994). Health and the social environment. *Environmental Impact Assessment Review, 14*, 359–375.

Samson, C. (1999). The physician and the patient. In C. Samson (Ed.), *Health studies, a critical and cross cultural reader*. United Kingdom: Blackwell Publishers.

Sanjek, R. (1990). On ethnographic validity. In R. Sanjek (Ed.), *Fieldnotes, the makings of anthropology*. Ithaca and London: Cornell University Press

Saradama, R. D., Higginbotham, N., & Nitcher, M. (2000). Social factors influencing the acquisition of antibiotic use in Kerala State, South India. *Social Science and Medicine, 50*(6), 891–903.

Saris, J. A. (1995). Telling stories: Life histories, illness narratives and institutional landscapes. *Culture, Medicine and Psychiatry, 19*, 39–72.

Seal, S. C. (1971). *An introduction to hospital-patient relationship*. Kolkata: Nababharat Publishers.

Sen, A. (2002). Health perception versus observation: Self-reported morbidities have severe limitations and can be extremely misleading. *BMJ, 324*, 360–361.

Shah, G. (1997). *Public health and urban development: The plague in Surat*. New Delhi: Sage Publications.

Shiva, M. (1985). Towards a healthy use of pharmaceuticals: An Indian perspective. *Development Dialogue, 2*, 69–93.

Singh, D. (2001). Clouds of cholera and clouds around cholera. In D. Kumar (Ed.), *Disease and medicine in India*. India History Congress: New Delhi.

Smith, D. C. (1981). Medical science, medical practice and the emerging concept of typhus in mid-eighteenth century Britain. In W. F. Bynum & V. Nutton (Eds.), *Theories of fever from antiquity to enlightenment*. Medical History Supplement No. 1, London: Wellcome Institute for the History of Medicine.

Smith, W. D. (1981). Implicit fever theory in epidemics 5 and 7. In W. F. Bynum & V. Nutton (Eds.), *Theories of fever from antiquity to enlightenment*. Medical History Supplement No. 1, London: Wellcome Institute for the History of Medicine.

Spradley, J. P. (1980). *Participant observation*. Australia and United Kingdom: Wadsworth, Thomson Learning.

Steele, J. L., & McBroom, W. H. (1972). Conceptual and empirical dimensions of health behaviour. *Journal of Health and Social Behaviour, 13*, 382–393.

Suchman, E. A. (1963). *Sociology and the field of public health*. New York: Russell Sage Foundation.

Sujatha, V. (2014). *Sociology of health and medicine: New perspectives*. Oxford: Oxford University Press.

Sushama, P. N. (1990). Social context of health behavior in Kerala. In J. F. Caldwell, S. Findley & P. Caldwell et al. (Eds.), *What we know about health transition: The cultural, social and behavioral determinants of health* (Vol. II). Canberra Australia: Australia National University Printing Service for the Health Transition Centre.

Temkin, O. (1964). Historical aspects of drug therapy. In P. Talaly (Ed.), *Drugs in our society*. Baltimore: Johns Hopkins University.

Thankappan, K. R. (2001). Some health implications of globalization in Kerala, India. *Bulletin of the World Health Organization, 79*(9), 892.

Tharamangalam, J. (1998). The perils of social development without economic growth: The development debacle of Kerala, India. *Bulletin of Concerned Asian Scholars, 30*(1), 23–34.

The Hindu, October 18, 2006: *Myths prevail in society about dengue*.

Thorn, G. W., Adams, R. D., Braunwald, E., Isselbacher, K. J., & Petersdorf, R. G. (Eds.). *Harrison's principles of internal medicine* (7th ed., pp. 48–62). New Delhi: Tata McGraw Hill.

Trenn, T. J. (1981). Ludwick Fleck's 'on the question of the foundation of medical knowledge'. *Journal of Medicine and Philosophy, 6*, 237–256.

Trostle, J. A. (2005). *Epidemiology and culture*. New York: Cambridge University Press.

Tuckett, D. (1976). Doctors and patients. In David Tuckett (Ed.), *An introduction to medical sociology*. London: Tavistock.

Turner, B. S. (2000). The history of the changing concepts of health and illness: Outline of a general model of illness categories. In G. Albrecht, R. Fitzpatrick, & S. Schrimshaw (Eds.), *Handbook of social studies in health and medicine*. London: Sage.

Varatharajan, D., Sadanandan, R., Thankappan, R. et al. (2002). *Idle capacity in resource strapped Government Hospitals in Kerala, size, distribution and determining factors*. Thiruvananthapuram, Kerala: Achuta Menon Centre for Health Science Studies, Sri Chitra Tirunal Institute of Medical Sciences and Technology.

Vinayachandran, P. (2001). *Kerala Chikilsa Charithram (Malayalam: Study) history of medical care in Kerala*. Kollam: Current Books.

Vishwanathan, S. (1997). *A carnival for science, essays on science, technology and development*. Calcutta, New Delhi: Oxford University Press.

Waitzkin, H. (1979). Medicine, superstructure and micropolitics. *Social Science and Medicine, 13A*, 601–619.

Waitzkin, H. (1981). The social origins of illness—A neglected history. *International Journal of Health Services, 11*, 77–103.

Ward, H., Mertens, T., & Thomas, C. (1997). Health-seeking behaviour and the control of sexually transmitted disease. *Health Policy and Planning, 12*(1), 19–28.

Weiss, M. (2001). Cultural epidemiology: An introduction and overview. *Anthropology and Medicine, 8*(1), 1–29.

White, K. (2002). *An introduction to the sociology of health and illness.* London: Sage.

Wintrobe, M. M., Thorn, G. W., Adams, R. D., Braunwald, E., Isselbacher, K. J., & Petersdorf, R. G. (Eds.). (1974). *Harrison's principles of internal medicine* (7th ed.). New Delhi: Tata McGraw Hill.

Wright, P., & Treacher, A. (Eds.) *The problem of medical knowledge: Examining social construction of medicine.* Edinburgh: Edinburgh University Press.

Wulff, H. R. (1990). Function and value of medical knowledge in modern diseases. In H. A. Ten Have, G. K. Kimsam, & S. F. Spicher (Eds.), *The growth of medical knowledge.* London: Kluwer Academic Publishers.

Yardley, L. (Ed.). (1997). *Material discourses of health and illness.* London: Routledge.

Young, A. (1981). The creation of medical knowledge, some problems in interpretation. *Social Science and Medicine, 15B*, 376–386.

Young, A. (1982). The anthropologies of illness and sickness. *Annual Review of Anthropology, 11*, 257–285.

Zola, I. K. (1972). Medicine as an institution of social control. *Sociological Review, 20*, 487–503.